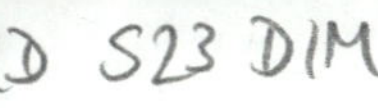

Maxillofacial Injuries

Maxillofacial Injuries

A Synopsis of Basic Principles, Diagnosis and Management

George Dimitroulis, MDSc (Melb.), FDSRCS (Eng.), FFDRCS (Irl.)
Formerly Clinical Fellow in Oral and Maxillofacial Surgery, College of Dentistry, University of Florida, USA

Brian Avery FRCS (Edin.), FDSRCS (Eng.)
Consultant Oral and Maxillofacial Surgeon, Middlesbrough General Hospital, UK

wright

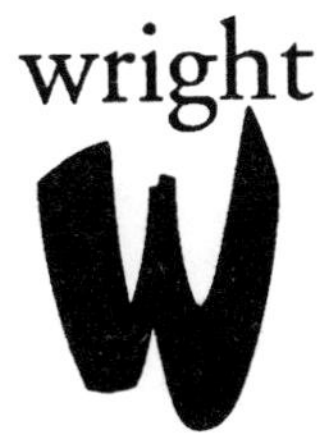

Wright
An imprint of Butterworth-Heinemann
Linacre House, Jordan Hill, Oxford OX2 8DP
A division of Reed Educational and Professional Publishing Ltd

A member of the Reed Elsevier plc group

OXFORD BOSTON JOHANNESBURG
MELBOURNE NEW DELHI SINGAPORE

First Published 1994
Reprinted 1996

British Library Cataloguing in Publication Data
Dimitroulis, George
Maxillofacial Injuries: A Synopsis of Basic Principles, Diagnosis and Management
I. Title II. Avery, Brian
617.52044

ISBN 0 7236 1010 X

Typeset by Keytec Typesetting Ltd, Bridport, Dorset
Printed and bound in Great Britain by Biddles Ltd, Guildford and King's Lynn

Contents

Preface

Over the years there have been numerous textbooks on the subject of maxillofacial injuries, some of which have become the backbone of this specialised field of surgery. It is a fact, however, that many great works on maxillofacial injuries have either been expensive or in the case of smaller books have had a limited scope.

The fundamental aim of this handbook is to present a comprehensive synopsis of all aspects of maxillofacial trauma in a clear, concise and orderly manner that will hopefully appeal not only to those who are revising for examinations, but also to the casual reader seeking a reminder to the field of maxillofacial trauma.

Although the bulk of this book is pitched at the individual in surgical training, there are nonetheless a substantial number of sections which undergraduates in dentistry and medicine may find extremely useful and hence act as a bridge between major works in this field and undergraduate teaching.

Each chapter follows a general sequence of surgical anatomy, classification of injuries, clinical presentation, investigations, treatment options and associated complications.

It is not the intention of this small handbook to cover all aspects of maxillofacial injuries in great detail, hence many points have merely been listed for completeness. The authors hope that this book will fulfil the essential needs of those with more than just a fleeting interest in the field of maxillofacial injuries.

George Dimitroulis
Brian Avery

Chapter 1

Introduction

Basic principles

Facial fractures versus other fractures

Facial fractures differ from fractures of other bones in the human skeleton in three important ways:

1. Risk to the airway – directly compromised
2. Presence of teeth – assists with stabilising fractures
3. Excellent blood supply of facial bones – promotes rapid healing

Fracture types seen in all bones

1. Simple – displaced/non-displaced
2. Compound – exposed bone or involvement of teeth
3. Comminuted – multiple fragments
4. Complicated – e.g. involving nerves, vessels, pleura, etc.
5. Greenstick – bending and splintering of bone in children
6. Pathological – e.g. cyst or tumour

Fracture dynamics of bones generally

The degree of fracture displacement will depend on:

1. Degree of force
2. Direction of force
3. Point of impact
4. Type of injury – blunt or sharp
5. Attached muscles – particularly important in mandibular fractures

Healing of bone

The following is the basic sequence of events when a bone heals:

1. Haemorrhage

2. Inflammation
3. Haematoma – organisation of blood clot and ingrowth of granulation tissue
4. Provisional callus:
   a. Osteoid – protein matrix with initial calcification 6–7 days
   b. Woven bone – irregular bridging trabeculae 2–3 weeks
5. Definitive callus – Lamellar bone 4–5 weeks
6. Remodelling:
   a. Resorption/deposition
   b. Compact bone – Haversian system

Factors which delay healing

Local

- Infection
- Foreign bodies
- Mobility
- Poor vascularity – irradiation

Systemic

- Increasing age
- Disease – e.g. diabetes
- Drugs – e.g. steroids
- Deficiency – e.g. malnutrition

Clinical features of maxillofacial injuries

Aetiology

1. Assaults – most common in western society
2. Road traffic accidents – most common in developing nations
3. Sports injuries
4. Falls
5. Industrial accidents

Predisposing factors

1. Alcohol
2. Epilepsy
3. Bone pathology – e.g. cysts, tumours

Presentation

1. Pain
2. Swelling
3. Loss of function – e.g. trismus, limited eye movement causing diplopia
4. Malocclusion
5. Altered sensation – nerve damage

Background

1. Time of injury
2. Mode of injury
3. Loss of consciousness
4. Treatment prior to admission

Medical history

1. Allergies
2. Drugs – e.g. insulin, steroids, anticoagulants
3. Illnesses – past and present
4. Previous surgery
5. Smoking and alcohol intake

General assessment

1. Airway
2. Shock
3. Haemorrhage
4. Level of consciousness
5. Overt infection

Clinical examination

1. Lacerations
2. Swelling
3. Ecchymosis
4. Visible or palpable deformity
5. Abnormal mobility and crepitus
6. Palpable tenderness
7. Impaired function – e.g. trismus, diplopia
8. Malocclusion
9. Nerve injury

Radiographic investigations of maxillofacial injuries

Plain X-rays must be taken in at least two planes at right angles to each other.

Standard projections

Orbits and Antra

- Occipito-mental 15 and 30 degrees

Maxillary bones

- Occipito-mental 15 and 30 degrees
- Lateral skull

Malar bones

- Occipito-mental 15 and 30 degrees
- Submento-vertical

Mandible

- Postero-anterior of mandible
- Orthopantomogram
- Right and left lateral obliques

Frontal bones

- Occipito-mental 15 and 30 degrees
- Lateral skull
- Brow-up lateral skull

Other projections sometimes used

- Dental/intraoral films
- Tangential skull views – soft tissues for emphysema or a foreign body
  – depressed fractures
- Transcranial and transpharyngeal views of temporomandibular joint
- CT scans – complex midface fracture, e.g. naso-ethmoidal fractures
  – three-dimensional reconstruction
  – coronal views for blowout fractures

Other important X-rays

- Cervical spine – to show fractures:
  Lateral
  Transoral view of odontoid peg
- Chest – for chest injury or aspiration:
  Postero-anterior
  Lateral

Principles of management

Preliminary treatment

1. Establish and maintain AIRWAY
2. Establish that patient is BREATHING – intubate if necessary
3. Arrest HAEMORRHAGE (shock rarely present if facial injuries only)
4. Examination of injuries
5. Temporary immobilisation of suspected fractures
6. Infection – prophylaxis
7. Pain relief – avoid sedation

Treatment priorities

Immediate intervention

1. Respiratory obstruction
2. Cardiac arrest
3. Massive bleeding

Treatment required urgently

1. Intra-abdominal bleeding
2. Head injuries – significant head injuries
   – deterioration
3. Chest injuries
4. Compound fractures of limbs

Treatment that can wait

Maxillofacial trauma

Treatment of soft tissue injuries

1. Tetanus prophylaxis
2. Antibiotics

3. Irrigation
4. Debridement – removal of severely contused tissue and foreign bodies
5. Haemostasis
6. Primary closure – accurately approximate freshened wound edges with careful suturing to minimise scarring
7. Skin loss – avoid secondary healing of facial wounds:
   a. Undermine skin edges and advance
   b. Skin grafts
   c. Local flaps
   d. Suture skin to oral mucosa – gunshot wounds

General principles of fracture treatment

1. **Debridement**
2. **Reduction**
   a. Closed manipulation
   b. Traction
   c. Open reduction
3. **Fixation**
   a. External:
      i. external pin fixation
      ii. halo frames
   b. Internal:
      i. non-rigid:
         suspension wiring
         circum-mandibular wiring
         transosseous wiring
         intramedullary pins
      ii. rigid:
         adaptational – plates or bicortical screws
         compression – plates or lag screws
4. **Immobilisation**
   Intermaxillary fixation
5. **Functional rehabilitation**

Specific injuries requiring specialist attention

1. Eyes and eyelids
2. Nasolacrimal apparatus – severed ends must be realigned and splinted internally with fine silastic tubing
3. Parotid duct – alignment and suturing

4. Facial nerve – repair in case of proximal injuries
5. Bites – human bites have high infection rates and should only be loosely sutured
6. Gunpowder and grease injuries

Complications of maxillofacial trauma

Adverse healing of fractures

Malunion

Malaligned healing of fractures due to inadequate reduction, possible osteotomy required to correct.

Delayed union

Disturbed and prolonged healing, e.g. resulting from localised and systemic fractures.

Nonunion

No bony healing.

Compromised airway

Causes

1. Trismus
2. Gross oedema – especially tongue and floor of mouth
3. Intermaxillary fixation
4. Lying on back – allows tongue to obstruct oropharynx
5. Aspiration of loose debris and tooth segments
6. Blocked nasal or oropharyngeal tubes

Management of compromised airway

1. Patient positioning:
   a. Conscious – sitting up and leaning forwards
   b. Unconscious – recovery position with chin lift
2. Airways – oropharyngeal or nasopharyngeal tubes
3. Endotracheal tube
4. Cricothyroidotomy – for complete airway obstruction
5. Tracheostomy – especially with chest and head injuries

Infection

Causes of fracture site infection

1. Compound injury
2. Foreign bodies
3. Devitalised teeth
4. Pre-existing oral infection – e.g. pericoronitis
5. Immunocompromised patient – e.g. diabetes, steroids, anaemia
6. Radiotherapy – previous treatment

Antibiotic therapy in maxillofacial trauma

Antibiotic prophylaxis is often important in maxillofacial injuries. Suggested antibiotic regimen:

- Intraoral breach – penicillin and metronidazole
- Skin – flucloxacillin/cephalosporin
- Contaminated wound – penicillin and metronidazole
- CSF leak – antibiotics which cross blood–brain barrier, i.e. sulphadimidine, septrin, cephalosporin

Further reading

Bramley P. (1985). Basic principles of treatment. In *Maxillofacial Injuries* vol. 1 (Rowe N.L. and Williams J.Ll., eds). Edinburgh: Churchill Livingstone, chap. 2.

Brook I.M. and Wood M. (1983). Aetiology and incidence of facial fractures in adults. *Int. J. Oral Surg.* **12**, 293.

Frame J.W. and Wake M.J. (1982). Evaluation of maxillofacial injuries by use of computerized tomography. *J. Oral Maxillofac. Surg.* **40**, 482.

Helfrick J.F. (1991). Early assessment and treatment planning of the maxillofacial trauma patient. In *Oral and Maxillofacial Trauma* vol. 1 (Fonseca R.J. and Walker R.V., eds). Philadelphia: W.B. Saunders, chap. 13.

Leigh J.M., Garfield J., Rowe N.L., and Williams J.Ll. (1985). Primary care. In *Maxillofacial Injuries* vol. 1 (Rowe N.L. and Williams J.Ll., eds). Edinburgh: Churchill Livingstone, chap. 3.

Rowe N.L. (1969). Non-union of the mandible and maxilla. *J. Oral Surg.*, **27**, 520.

Chapter 2

Dentoalveolar injuries

Applied dental anatomy

Enamel – ceramic nature, very brittle.
Dentine – ceramic but with a certain degree of viscoelasticity.
Pulp – no resistance to physical trauma. It is the tissue essential for tooth vitality and contains vascular, nervous, reparative and odontogenic elements.
Periodontal membrane – a hammock of collagen fibres that support the tooth within its bony socket. Its hydroelastic properties function as a buffer between tooth and socket during functional loading of teeth.
Alveolar bone – high degree of organic matrix and is capable of small amount of distortion before fracture.

Epidemiology

The most frequently fractured teeth are upper central incisors followed by lateral incisors. Most are single tooth injuries which are more often displaced rather than fractured. Multiple tooth injuries commonly present with extensive crown and root fractures.

Predisposing factors

- Male > female
- Malocclusion – class II division I
- Contact sports
- Interpersonal violence
- Leisure activities, e.g. cycling, skateboarding
- Handicaps
- Falls, e.g. epilepsy

Classification

Tooth fractures

1. **Uncomplicated crown fractures**:
   a. Enamel – including cracks
   b. Enamel and dentine (Figure 2.1(a))
      i. supragingival
      ii. subgingival
2. **Complicated crown fractures (involving the pulp)**:
   a. Horizontal
      i. supragingival (Figure 2.1(b))
      ii. subgingival
   b. Diagonal
      i. supragingival
      ii. subgingival (Figure 2.1(c))
   c. Vertical
3. **Root fractures** (Figure 2.2):
   a. Apical third
   b. Middle third
   c. Coronal third

Periodontal injuries

1. **Concussion** – compression injury to periodontal membrane with tooth retained in original position

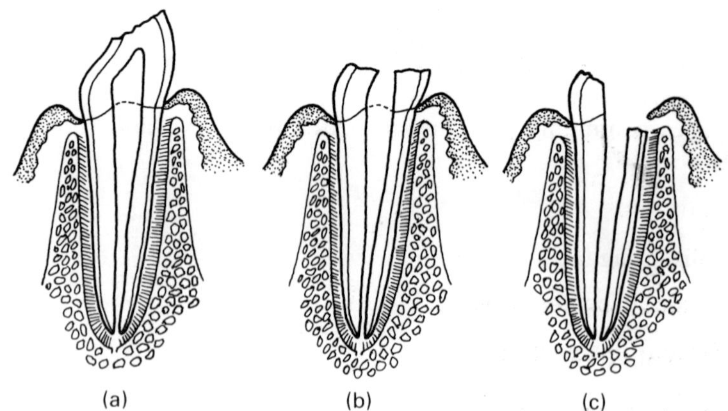

Figure 2.1 (a) Fracture of enamel of incisal edge exposing dentine. (b) Supragingival fracture of crown exposing both dentine and pulp. (c) Subgingival fracture of crown and part of root, exposing the dentine pulp and periodontal membrane.

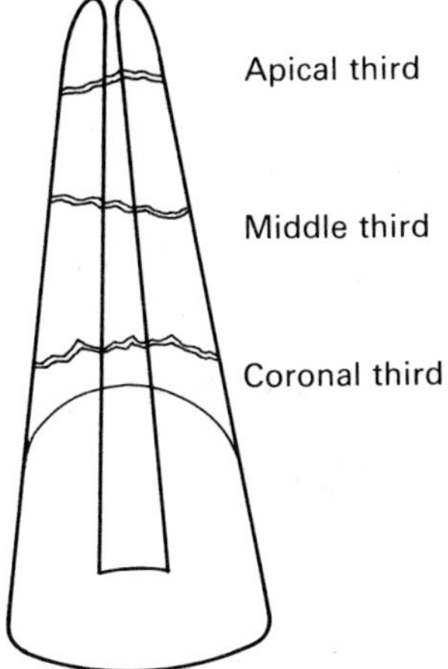

Figure 2.2 Root fractures.

2. **Subluxation** – tooth partially displaced from socket without injury to socket walls
3. **Displacement** – tooth partially displaced from socket with associated injury to alveolar walls
4. **Avulsion** – complete loss of tooth from socket

Alveolar bone injuries

1. Crushing or compression associated with tooth displacements
2. Fracture of alveolar wall
3. Fracture of alveolar process
4. Fracture of maxilla or mandible

Injuries to the gingivae

1. Contusion
2. Abrasion
3. Laceration

Combinations of the above

Clinical assessment

Presenting complaint

1. Tooth sensitive to hot and cold
2. Sharp tooth

3. Mobile tooth/teeth
4. Oral pain
5. Oral bleeding
6. Malocclusion

Background

1. Cause
2. Time of accident
3. Any treatment prior to presentation, i.e. reimplanted tooth
4. Loss of consciousness
5. All missing dental fragments accounted for? – Chest X-ray
6. Tetanus status?

Clinical assessment

1. Check for head injury
2. Lacerations to face or scalp
3. Check for fractured jaws
4. Lips – swelling, laceration, embedded foreign or dental fragments
5. Oral mucosa – haematoma, lacerations
6. Teeth – missing, displaced, fractured, mobile, exposed pulps, bleeding gingivae

Investigations

1. **X-rays**:
   a. Dental – periapicals, occlusals
   b. Orthopantomogram – jaw fractures
   c. Soft tissue of lips – foreign bodies, tooth fragments
   d. Chest X-rays – aspirated tooth or tooth fragment?
2. **Vitality test** – Early results usually equivocal so it is best to retest at later date, e.g. 2 months, prior to commencement of root canal treatment
3. **Transillumination** – To demonstrate cracks of enamel

Treatment

Uncomplicated crown fractures

1. **Enamel cracks** – no immediate treatment usually needed but careful follow-up for tooth vitality is important

2. **Enamel fracture** – relief of sharpness, restoration, recement fragment if possible
3. **Enamel and dentine** – relief of sharpness, protect dentine with lining and semipermanent restoration or recement fragment, follow-up vitality of tooth prior to permanent restoration

Complicated crown fractures

1. **Supragingival** – direct pulp capping or partial pulpotomy, dentine lining, temporary or semipermanent restoration or recement missing fragment if possible, follow-up vitality of tooth prior to root canal treatment and permanent restoration, e.g. crown
2. **Subgingival** – as for supragingival fractures but may need to orthodontically extrude root to facilitate permanent restoration. Extraction of tooth may be necessary
3. **Vertical fractures** – usually extraction necessary

Root fractures

1. **Apical third** – if root canal treatment is required then treat only up to fracture line
2. **Middle third** – doubtful prognosis but retain if possible
3. **Coronal third** – consider orthodontically extruding root, otherwise extraction necessary

Periodontal injuries

A. Subluxation and displacement

Manipulate tooth back into correct position (may require local anaesthesia), and splint to adjacent teeth if necessary for between 4 days and 4 weeks depending on degree of stability after reduction

B. Tooth avulsions

The prognosis of an avulsed tooth depends on the viability of its periodontal membrane which is in turn dependent on the period in which the tooth remains out of its socket and the storage medium used prior to reimplantation

1. **Telephone advice**:
   a. Rinse tooth in water
   b. Replace immediately with light finger pressure

   c. If unable to replace tooth store in milk or place in 'cling film'
   d. Attend dental surgery immediately
2. **At the clinic**:
   a. Irrigate tooth socket with saline to remove blood clots
   b. Gently reimplant tooth with digital pressure, avoid touching root surface
   c. Splint to adjacent teeth for approximately 4 weeks
   d. Relieve tooth from occlusion
   e. Antibiotics
   f. Commence root canal therapy between 7 and 14 days
   g. Advise soft diet
3. **Long-term follow-up**:
   a. Review at regular intervals with serial radiographs
   b. Check for either inflammatory root resorption or replacement root resorption and subsequent ankylosis
   c. Rapid rejection of reimplanted tooth occurs with epithelial downgrowth
4. **Storage media for avulsed teeth**:
   a. Dry – 15 minutes
   b. Tap water – same as dry storage
   c. Normal saline – 2 hours
   d. Saliva – 2 hours
   e. Milk – 6 hours
   f. 'Cling film' – best storage medium

C. Notes on splinting of teeth

1. **Types of splints that can be used:**
   a. Aluminium foil
   b. Lead foil from dental X-ray films
   c. Cold-cure acrylic
   d. Interdental wiring
   e. Patients own mouthguard
   f. Etch bonded composite or glass ionomer
      i. non-reinforced – straight coverage or doughnut shaped
      ii. reinforced – wire
2. **Objectives of a splint**:
   a. Stabilize tooth/teeth after appropriate reduction
   b. Eliminate further damage and displacement
   c. Permit normal healing
3. **Requirements of a splint**:
   a. Must be readily and immediately available
   b. Atraumatic to tissues

c. Does not prevent diagnostic and follow-up treatment
d. Does not interfere with occlusion
e. Acceptable flexibility that permits physiological 'jiggling' movement of teeth in order to reduce likelihood of ankylosis
f. Permits maintenance of proper oral hygiene
g. Aesthetic appearance
h. Easily removed

Alveolar bone injuries

Principle same as other bone fractures:

1. Reduction – finger manipulation
2. Fixation – dental splints
3. Immobilisation – 4 weeks

Teeth within alveolar fragment act as excellent stabilising bone pins and can be anchored by a splint to adjacent teeth.

Antibiotics are advised.

Gingival injuries

Cover abrasions and other raw areas with antiseptic pack or 'coe-pak'.
Suture lacerations with 4/0 soluble sutures

Acute trauma of deciduous teeth

1. **Displacements** – intrusion or extrusion. Consider possible damage to underlying developing permanent tooth. Teeth should either be left or extracted
2. **Avulsion** – do not attempt to reimplant

Further reading

Andreasen J.O., and Andreasen F.M. (1990). *Essentials of Traumatic Injuries to the Teeth.* Copenhagen: Munksgaard.

Cvek M. (1978). A clinical report on partial pulpotomy and capping with calcium hydroxide in permanent incisors with complicated crown fracture. *J. Endodont.*, **4**, 232.

Hammarstrom L., Pierce A., Blomlof L., Feiglin B., and Lindskog S. (1986). Tooth avulsion and replantation – a review. *Endod. Dent. Traumatol.*, **2**, 1.

Chapter 3

Mandibular fractures

Surgical anatomy

Factors related to mandibular fractures

1. Prominent mandible
2. Fracture force – degree, direction, site of impact, sharp or blunt
3. Strength and resilience of mandible – generally speaking the mandible is strongest at point of the chin and weakens towards the condyles. Tensile strain is less resistant to fracture than compressive strain
4. Attached musculature – influences the **site** of fracture and **displacement** of fragments

Fracture sites (Figure 3.1)

1. Multiple fractures > single fractures
2. Symphysis – thickest and strongest area. Fractures are frequently parasymphyseal and rarely occur in midline

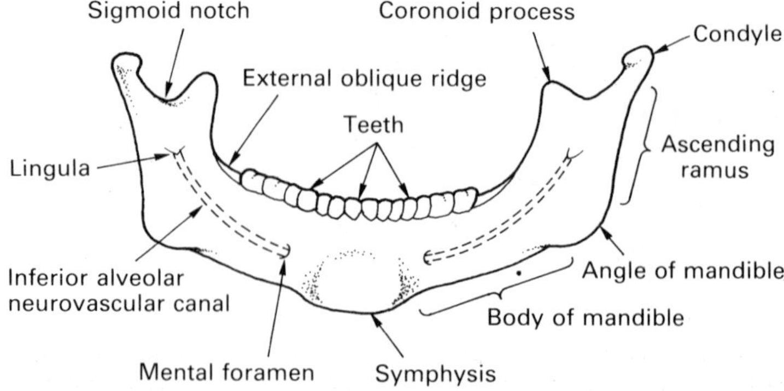

Figure 3.1 Anatomy of the mandible (orthopantomogram projection).

3. Incisor region – fractures frequently oblique. Genial muscles displace fragments lingually. Mylohyoid muscle pulls fragments medially, so adjacent incisor teeth overlap
4. Canine region – point of weakness associated with long canine tooth
5. Angle region – fractures here may result from indirect force:
   a. Weakness due to right angle between body and ramus and also presence of wisdom tooth
   b. Strength – due to pterygomasseteric sling
   c. Displacement – due to opposing effects of pterygomasseteric sling and suprahyoid musculature (Figure 3.2)
6. Inferior dental bundle – fibrous sheath provides support and protection for vessels and nerve. This accounts for the low incidence of permanent nerve damage after fracture between mandibular foramen and mental foramen
7. Combination fractures – e.g. Guardsman fracture consisting of symphyseal fracture plus both condylar necks OR body fracture on one side and condylar neck on other side

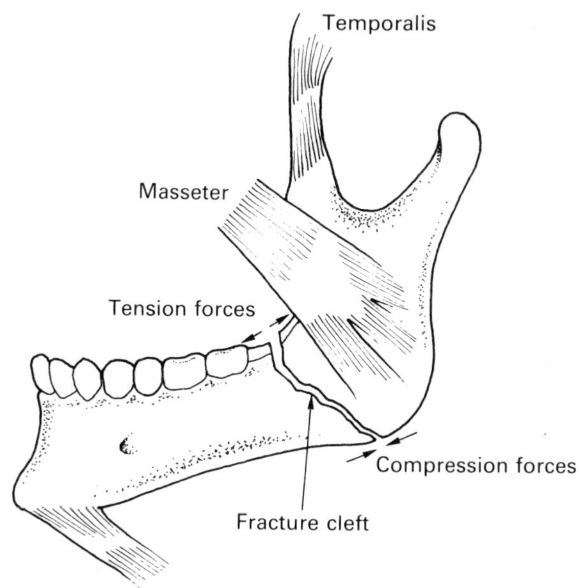

Figure 3.2 The pull of the surrounding musculature results in compression forces at the lower border and tension forces at the upper border of a fracture through the angle of the mandible.

Fracture healing and blood supply to mandible

1. Multifactorial blood supply:
   a. Endosteal – inferior dental artery
   b. Periosteal – facial, lingual, buccal and mylohyoid arteries
   c. Muscles – genial muscles at symphysis, pterygomasseteric sling and temporalis muscle at ramus
2. Healing potential:
   a. Endosteal supply to body of mandible decreases with increasing age
   b. Atrophic edentulous mandibles receive only periosteal blood supply. If it is stripped for plating may result in non-union of fractures
   c. Stripping pterygomasseteric sling off ramus may result in avascular necrosis

Classification

1. **Anatomical** (Figure 3.3):

Condylar neck	35%
Angle	20%
Body	20%
Parasymphysis	13%
Symphysis	11%
Coronoid	1%

2. **Potential**
   - Horizontally favourable or unfavourable
   - Vertically favourable or unfavourable

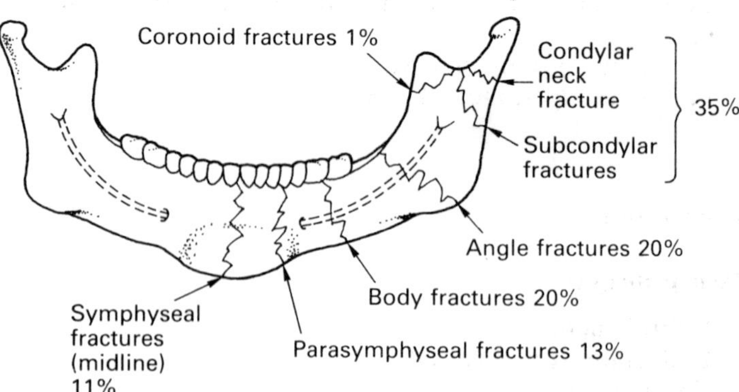

Figure 3.3 Mandibular fractures described by anatomical site. Note: angle and body fractures involve the inferior alveolar neurovascular canal.

3. **Dental**
   - Class I – teeth present on both sides of fracture line
   - Class II – teeth on one side of fracture line
   - Class III – no teeth present on either fragment

Clinical features

Signs and symptoms

1. Lacerations – bleeding
2. Swelling
3. Ecchymosis – sublingual haematoma signifies fracture of lingual plate
4. Visible and palpable deformity of bone
5. Abnormal mobility and crepitus of mandible
6. Malocclusion and step deformity of teeth
7. Palpable tenderness
8. Inferior dental nerve disruption – paraesthesia or anaesthesia of lower lip
9. Damaged teeth – loose or missing including missing fragments
10. Bleeding from ear – tear of skin of external auditory meatus due to anatomical proximity of mandibular condyle

Teeth in fracture line

Potential impediment to healing because of infection:

1. Compound fracture into mouth via open periodontal membrane
2. Tooth may become non-vital
3. Pre-existing periodontal disease

Treatment

Basic principles

1. Debridement
2. Reduction – open/closed
3. Fixation – internal/external
4. Immobilisation
5. Functional rehabilitation

Intermaxillary fixation (Figure 3.4)

This is a form of immobilisation which stabilises bone fragments in a blind manner, sometimes resulting in non-precise anatomical alignment and prolonged secondary bone healing with large callus formation.

1. Eyelet wiring
2. Arch bars
3. Cast-cap silver splints
4. Gunning splints

External pin fixation

Bone pins (Moule, Toller) inserted transcutaneously into main anterior and posterior fragments and joined by universal joints and connecting rods or plastic splints.

Advantages

a. Discontinuity defects – tumour resection, avulsive trauma, to maintain major fragments in correct anatomical position prior to bone grafting
b. Pathological fractures
c. Gunshot injuries
d. Infected fracture sites

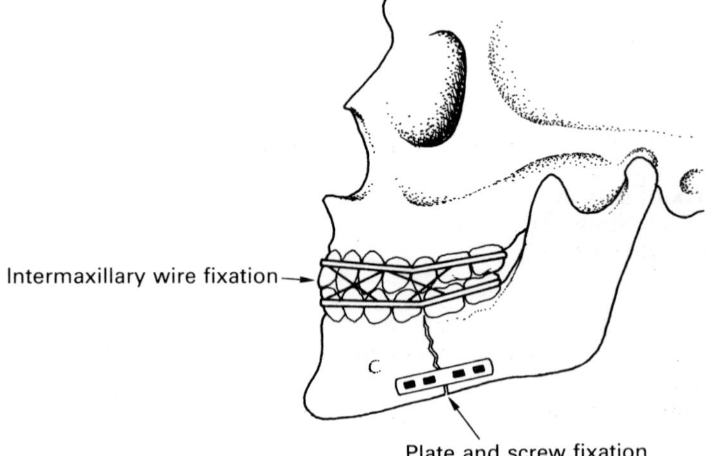

Figure 3.4 Two methods of treatment for a fracture through the body of the mandible.

Disadvantages
a. Non-precise anatomical alignment
b. Restricts patient activity because of risk of knock to pins
c. Infection and scarring around pin sites
d. Insertion of pin into inferior dental nerve – paraesthesia or anaesthesia

Internal fixation

Permits more precise anatomical reduction:

1. Transosseous wiring – upper border, lower border or mid-body
2. Intramedullary pins – Kirschner wire/Steinmann pin
3. Rigid internal fixation (Figure 3.4):
   a. adaptational – plates, titanium mesh, bicortical screws
   b. compression – plates, lag screws

Transosseous wires

Advantages
a. Permits precise anatomical bone reduction
b. Fairly easy to apply
c. Increased stability

Disadvantages
a. Poor rigidity and directional control – very little wire/bone contact
b. Often requires additional intermaxillary fixation
c. Wire may pull out from bone leading to delayed or poor bone healing

Intramedullary pins

Advantages
a. Rapid stabilisation of bone fragments
b. For reducing displaced condylar fractures when surgery necessary
c. Limited operating time, e.g. very sick patient

Disadvantages
a. Difficult to use in oblique fractures
b. Fractures may displace around long axis of pin
c. Requires intermaxillary fixation

Rigid internal fixation (see Chapter 5)

The use of plates and screws in the direct fixation of fractures

Advantages

a. Permits primary bone healing
b. Increased three-dimensional, mechanical and functional stability
c. Precise anatomical reduction and enhanced bone healing
d. No additional fixation required
e. Greater patient comfort – function restored early
f. Intermaxillary fixation not needed – airway maintained and patient can eat

Disadvantages

a. Stress-shielding
b. Expense
c. May interfere with CT scans and radiotherapy
d. Intermaxillary fixation may be necessary as well
e. Risk of screws damaging inferior dental nerve or teeth
f. Infection may necessitate removal of plate
g. Wound dehiscence

Metallic mesh implants or trays

a. Much thinner than bone plates with greater surface area
b. Adaptable internal rigid fixation used for treatment of:
   i. Non-unions
   ii. Discontinuity defects – holds bone grafts, ideally of cancellous bone

Teeth in fracture line

Management

1. X-rays (including periapical radiographs – usually only to establish fracture of tooth when in doubt)
2. Antibiotics
3. Follow-up with immediate extraction if infection ensues

Removal of teeth in fracture line

1. Infected fracture sites
2. Subluxed tooth
3. Fractured tooth root

4. Pre-existing periapical or gingival infection
5. Advanced caries

Postoperative care

Immediate

1. Monitor vital signs – temperature, blood pressure, pulse, respiratory rate
2. Soft diet and good oral hygiene – liquid diet necessary if intermaxillary fixation present
3. Monitor fluid balance
4. Analgesics, antibiotics
5. Post-reduction X-rays

Late

1. Testing of union and removal of intermaxillary fixation if present
2. Occlusal adjustment – with elastic intermaxillary fixation if necessary
3. Monitor recovery of nerve dysfunction and vitality of teeth
4. Encourage jaw function

Complications

Preoperative complications

1. Risk to airway
2. Bleeding
3. Displacement of loose fragments – into soft tissues or aspiration of teeth

Intraoperative problems

1. Nerve damage
2. Inadequate fracture reduction
3. Access difficulty, e.g. placing of plate across angle fracture

Postoperative complications

1. Infection/wound dehiscence
2. Malocclusion

3. Malunion, delayed union, or non-union
4. Temporomandibular joint derangement
5. Non-vital teeth – infection
6. Problems with fixation

Management of atrophic edentulous mandible

- Ideally open reduction and internal fixation
- If possible, two plates should be applied supraperiosteally near lower border
- In event of non-union consider freshening bone ends and a bone graft in a rigidly fixed titanium mesh tray as the probable best form of treatment

Further reading

Amaratunga N.A.deS. (1988). A comparative study of the clinical aspects of edentulous and dentulous mandibular fractures. *J. Oral Maxillofac. Surg.*, **46**, 3.

Banks P. (1991). *Killey's Fractures of the Mandible* 3rd edn. Oxford: Butterworth-Heinemann (Wright).

Bradley J.C. (1972). Age changes in the vascular supply of the mandible. *Br. Dent. J.* **132**, 142.

Bruce R., and Fonseca R.J. (1991). Mandibular fractures. In *Oral and Maxillofacial Trauma* (Fonseca R.J. and Walker R.V., eds). Philadelphia: W. B. Saunders.

Ellis E., Moos K.F. and El-Attar A. (1985). Ten years of mandibular fractures – an analysis of 2137 cases. *Oral Surg. Oral Med. Oral Pathol.*, **59**, 120.

Gariulo E.A. (1973). Use of titanium mesh and autogenous bone marrow in the repair of a non-united mandibular fracture; report of a case and review of the literature. *J. Oral Surg.*, **31**, 371.

Heslop I.H., Clarke P.B., Becker R., *et al.* (1985). Mandibular fractures: treatment by open reduction and direct skeletal fixation. In *Maxillofacial Injuries* vol. 1. (Rowe N.L. and Williams J.Ll., eds). Edinburgh: Churchill Livingstone, chap. 9.

Kahnberg K.E. and Ridell A. (1979). Prognosis of teeth involved in the fracture line. *Int. J. Oral Surg.* **8**, 163.

Morris J.H. (1949). Biphasic connector and external skeletal splint for the reduction and fixation of mandibular fractures. *Oral Surg. Oral Med. Oral Pathol.*, **2**, 1382.

Chapter 4

Condylar injuries

Categories of condylar injuries

1. **Contusion** – Injuries to the soft tissues around the joint or an effusion within the joint
2. **Dislocation** – Displacement of condylar head from glenoid fossa but still within capsule
3. **Fracture**
   a. Intracapsular – condylar head or neck
   b. Extracapsular – condylar neck or subcondylar

Classification of condylar fractures (Lindahl, 1977)

A. Fracture level (Figure 4.1)

1. Condylar head (intracapsular) – vertical, compression, comminuted
2. Condylar neck
3. Subcondylar

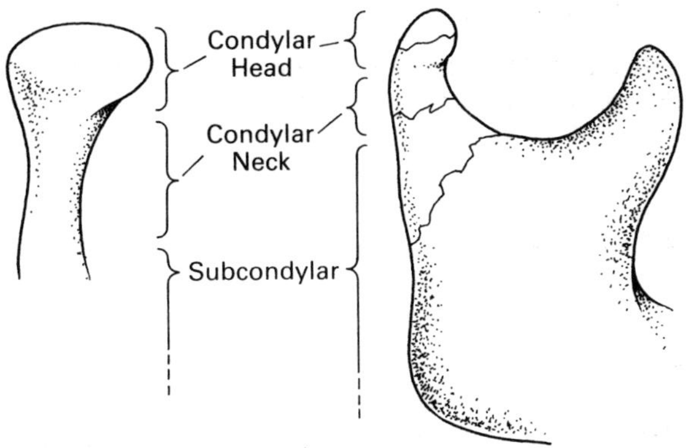

Figure 4.1 The three levels at which fractures of the mandibular condyle may occur.

B. Relation of condyle to mandible

1. Undisplaced – hairline fracture
2. Deviated
3. Displaced – medial or lateral overlap
4. Anterior/posterior overlap
5. No bony contact

C. Relation of condyle to glenoid fossa

1. Undisplaced
2. Displaced – condylar head still related to glenoid fossa
3. Dislocation – condylar head completely out of glenoid fossa. Condylar head usually lies anteromedial

Applied surgical anatomy

1. Usually indirect force
2. Medial displacement of condyles due to resistance of strong lateral ligaments
3. Deviation of mandible to injured side on opening due to loss of translatory movement
4. Narrow condylar neck and the elongated condylar head more likely to fracture than likelihood of penetration of condylar head through glenoid fossa into middle cranial fossa
5. Injuries to teeth more often seen with intracapsular trauma than subcondylar fractures
6. Condylar fractures more likely to occur with teeth apart and elevator muscles relaxed at time of injury
7. Trauma causes violent contraction of masticatory muscles resulting in a subcondylar fracture and anteromedial displacement of condyle
8. Trauma stimulates the trigeminal nerve supply of the temporomandibular joint which results in muscle spasm and restricted mobility

Clinical features

1. **Temporomandibular joint effusion/haemarthrosis**
   a. Ipsilateral posterior open-bite
   b. Midline shift to contralateral side
2. **Unilateral fracture**
   a. Ipsilateral premature contact posteriorly
   b. Ipsilateral midline shift

3. **Bilateral fracture dislocations**
   a. Anterior open-bite due to shortening of both mandibular rami
4. **Bilateral dislocation of condylar heads**
   a. Pseudoprognathism
   b. Inability to occlude teeth
   c. Elongated face
   d. Condyles palpable anterior to articular eminence with pre-auricular hollow

Treatment

Conservative

1. **Minimal displacement** – No active treatment. A normal occlusion is maintained which allows bony union to occur. In fracture-dislocation a functional pseudarthrosis may be produced
2. **Persistent malocclusion or severe pain** – A short period of intermaxillary fixation (7–10 days) until oedema and muscle spasm disappear
3. **Bilateral fractures** – A longer period of intermaxillary fixation (3–4 weeks) with posterior distraction blocks, e.g. gutta percha, acrylic wedges. Elastic traction may be necessary to close anterior open-bite

Surgical indications

1. Compound and comminuted fractures
2. Condylar displacements including fracture-dislocations with gross occlusal disruption, telescoping or mechanical interference
3. Multiple facial fractures where mandible is used to stabilise mid-face

Surgical approaches

1. Pre-auricular
2. Submandibular or retromandibular
3. Intraoral–difficult

Reduction

Difficult to re-position. Lateral pterygoid muscle may require detachment to allow reduction of fractured condyle. Sometimes condyle totally removed and re-positioned in glenoid fossa.

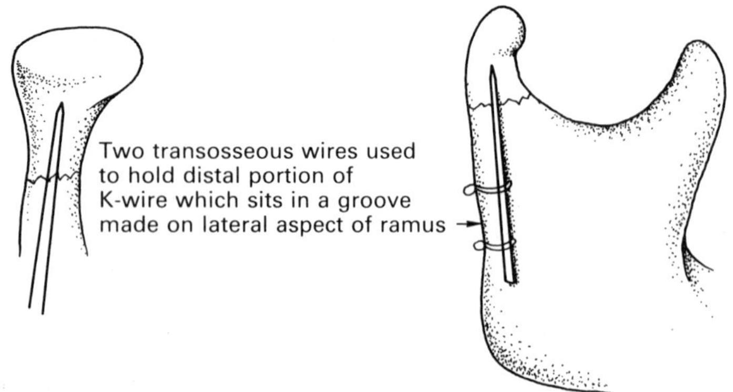

Figure 4.2 The use of a K-wire to skewer and fix a fractured condyle (Brown and Obeid 1984).

Fixation

1. Suture
2. Wires (Figure 4.2)
3. Plates
4. Pins – rarely

Conservative versus surgical treatment

1. Clinical data shows that bony union occurs after condylar fractures regardless of whether intermaxillary fixation is used or not
2. Studies on Rhesus monkeys found no difference between surgical and non-surgical treatment of condylar fractures

Specific management of special cases

Children under 12 years old

Bony union and remodelling of condylar head which is restored in the glenoid fossa occurs spontaneously in children. This ability to remodel declines after puberty.

1. Conservative non-immobilisation (most cases). Sometimes construction of a guide flange
2. Immobilisation less than 2 weeks – for gross displacement or a fracture when malocclusion may develop

3. Surgery – condylectomy for severe compound comminuted fractures which have a high risk of ankylosis. This can be followed by costochondral graft.

Temporomandibular joint contusion

Soft diet, analgesics and exercises when pain subsides. Bite-raising appliances may be used to distract the joints. Short-wave diathermy may help.

Compound fractures

Antibiotics, early surgical debridement and closure minimise the length of intermaxillary fixation. Encourage early function.

Penetration of glenoid fossa

This is a very rare injury.

1. Removal of condyle – open surgical procedure
2. Leave in situ – divide condyle at level of glenoid fossa with later joint reconstruction

Ramus and coronoid fractures

1. **Ramus fractures** – Exhibit very little displacement because of splinting action of pterygo-masseteric sling
2. **Coronoid fractures** – Only minimal displacement due to splinting action of tendinous insertion of temporalis muscle which is occasionally ruptured with elevation of tip into temporal fossa. No malocclusion but severe trismus. These fractures are rare because of protection afforded by overlying zygomatic arch and musculature. Coronoid process may fracture if injured when mouth open. More frequently, a fractured coronoid process is related to severe blunt trauma which damages overlying zygomatic arch, fractures the condyle and the coronoid process. In these circumstances patient may develop extra-articular ankylosis.

Complications of condylar injuries

1. **Temporomandibular joint pain/dysfunction syndrome** – Tearing and stretching of disc attachment may lead to this

2. **Disturbance in mandibular growth** – Condyle is site of secondary adaptation to demands of mandibular growth rather than a primary growth centre. It allows condylar head to remain in glenoid fossa as the mandible develops downwards and forwards – functional matrix theory
3. **Ankylosis** – Predisposing factors include:
   a. Children < 10 years old
   b. Intracapsular fractures
      i. Damaged meniscus – which acts as barrier to bony union
      ii. Comminuted head
      iii. Gross telescoping
   c. Lengthy periods of immobilisation, e.g. > 2 weeks
   d. Compound/comminuted fractures where coronoid and zygoma are involved
   e. Related to severe trauma – in the western world frequently seen after cycle accidents or a fall from a window

Treatment of dislocations

Acute dislocation

1. **Cause**
   a. Trauma
   b. Tooth extraction
   c. Habitual attention-seekers
   d. Drugs – with extrapyramidal effects, e.g. phenothiazines
   e. Spontaneous
2. **Treatment**
   a. Intracapsular local anaesthesia – to reduce reflex spasm of muscles of mastication
   b. Digital manipulation with or without sedation
   c. Reduction under general anaesthesia
   d. Instructions to avoid wide opening for 14 days

Chronic dislocations

1. **Less than 3 months**
   a. Manipulation – LA, sedation, GA with intermaxillary fixation for 14 days to allow healing
      i. Digital – downward and backward pressure with thumbs on posterior mandibular teeth
      ii. Wire traction or hooks at angles or coronoid process of mandible
      iii. Direct surgical exposure of joint

2. **Greater than 3 months**
   a. Condylotomy – closed or open approach
   b. Condylectomy
   c. Osteotomy – sagittal split, vertical subsigmoid

Recurrent dislocations

May be possible to prevent by eliminating predisposing factors, e.g. ill-fitting dentures or Class II malocclusion

1. **Tightening meniscus and capsule**
   a. Sclerosing agents – sodium tetradecyl sulphate (STD)
   b. Meniscal plication – fibrosis of lax ligaments
2. **Restricting condylar movements**
   a. Intermaxillary fixation
   b. Myotomy or condylotomy – rarely used
3. **Augmenting the eminence**
   a. Onlay grafts – bone from iliac crest
   b. Pins and screws inserted into eminence – loosen with time
   c. Dautrey procedure (Dautrey, 1975)
      i. Technique – downward displacement of zygomatic arch to obstruct movement of condylar head
      ii. Limitations
         Arch tends to fracture over age of 25
         Narrow bone of zygomatic arch may not provide sufficient obstruction to movement of condylar head – may be unreliable
   d. Downfracture of articular eminence – with interpositional graft
4. **Removing barriers that maintain dislocation**
   a. Eminectomy – good success but may lead to fibrosis
   b. High condylectomy – to facilitate return of condyle to fossa

Further reading

Banks P. (1991). *Killey's Fractures of the Mandible* 4th edn. Oxford: Butterworth-Heinemann (Wright).

Bradley P.F. (1985). *Maxillofacial Injuries* vol. 1 (Rowe N.L. and Williams J.LI., eds). Edinburgh: Churchill Livingstone, chap. 10.

Brown A.E. and Obeid G. (1984). A simplified method for the internal fixation of fractures of the mandibular condyle. *Br. J. Oral Maxillofac. Surg.*, **22**, 145.

Laskin D.M. (1978). The role of the meniscus in the etiology of post-traumatic temporomandibular joint ankylosis. *Int. J. Oral Surg.*, **7**, 340.

Lindahl L. (1977). Condylar fractures of the mandible. I. Classification and relation to age, occlusion and concomitant injuries of teeth and teeth-supporting structures and fractures of the mandibular body. *Int. J. Oral Surg.*, **6**, 12.

Lindahl L. (1977). Condylar fractures of the mandible. III. Positional changes of the chin. *Int. J. Oral Surg.*, **6**, 166.
Lindahl L. (1977). Condylar fractures of the mandible. IV. Function of the masticatory system. *Int. J. Oral Surg.*, **6**, 195.
Lindahl L. and Hollander L. (1977). Condylar fractures of the mandible. II. A radiographic study of remodelling process in the temporomandibular joint. *Int. J. Oral Surg.*, **6**, 153.
MacGregor A.B. and Fordyce G.L. (1957). The treatment of fractures of the neck of the mandibular condyle. *Br. Dent. J.*, **102**, 351.
Upton L.G. (1991). Management of injuries to the temporomandibular joint region. In *Oral and Maxillofacial Trauma* vol. 1 (Fonseca R.J. and Walker R.V., eds). Philadelphia: W.B. Saunders, chap. 17.
Walker R.V. (1960). Traumatic mandibular condylar fracture dislocations: effect on growth in the Macaca rhesus monkey. *Am. J. Surg.*, **100**, 850.
Zide M.F. and Kent J.N. (1983). Indications for open reduction of mandibular condylar fractures. *J. Oral Maxillofac. Surg.*, **41**, 89.

Chapter 5

Rigid internal fixation

Rigid internal fixation (RIF) refers to the direct fixation of fractures by plate and screw osteosynthesis, which has presently superseded other types of fixation for the management of facial fractures.

Historical

1920s – early use of rigid internal fixation (RIF) for mandibular fractures not encouraging
Roberts (1964) – adapted miniaturised orthopaedic plates for use in mandible
Brons and Boering (1970) – introduced lag screw fixation
Spiessl *et al.* (1972) – introduced use of compression plates and screws
Michelet *et al*. (1973) – transbuccal approach to screw placement
Champy *et al.* (1976) – miniaturised monocortical fixation placed along tension bands of mandible via intraoral approach

Advantages

1. **Primary bone healing**
   a. Rigid immobilisation
   b. Intimate contact
2. **Improved mechanical function and stability**
   Greater area of contact between bone and screw
3. **Direct and precise anatomical reduction**
   No need to distract fractures
4. **Less morbidity**
   a. No intermaxillary fixation
   b. Rapid return of jaw function and body weight
   c. Better oral hygiene
   d. Less postoperative discomfort

Indications

1. **Airway maintenance** – particularly in head injuries
2. **Early function**

RIF has superseded most other forms of fixation

Contraindications

1. **Contaminated fractures** – risk of infection
2. **Comminuted fractures** – difficult to plate multiple fragments
3. **Compound fractures** – where immediate or complete soft tissue cover is not possible
4. **Bone pathology**
5. **Young children** – presence of multiple unerupted teeth creates a problem of screw placement

Need for additional intermaxillary fixation

1. Associated condylar fractures which are not directly fixed
2. Associated midface fractures which are not internally fixed
3. Delay in treating fractures where an accurate reduction may not be possible – elastic traction may be required to gradually bring fragments together

Limitations

1. **Stress-shielding** – osteoporosis occurs under RIF which protects the fracture from normal functional forces of bone remodelling since forces are mediated via plate with higher modulus of elasticity
2. **Inflammation** – caused by:
   a. Metal corrosion
   b. Foreign body reaction
   c. Bone resorption around internally stressed appliances
3. **Interference** – radiotherapy, CT scans, MRI (titanium plates not usually a problem)
4. **Bulk**:
   a. Patient discomfort, e.g. plate at zygomatico-frontal suture – this can be overcome by using a low-profile plate or a microplate

   b. Interference with graft re-vascularisation
5. **Expense**

Complications

1. **Infection**
2. **Wound dehiscence**:
   a. Angle fracture where plate is just under mucosal incision on external oblique ridge
   b. Delay in treatment
   c. Poor oral hygiene
3. **Malocclusion**:
   a. Associated condylar fractures
   b. Compression plating – plate at lower border may cause occlusal separation
4. **Sensory disturbances**:
   a. Placement of screw in inferior dental canal
   b. Tissue retraction – injury to mental nerve
5. **Delayed union or non-union**

Failure of RIF

1. Inexperienced operator leading to poor technique
2. Delayed treatment leading to infection
3. Metal fatigue – leading to loose screws and fracture of plate
4. Wound dehiscence and exposure – immediate removal of hardware may be unnecessary if exposed site is kept clean and packed with antiseptic gauze

Removal of RIF

1. **Clinical indications**:
   a. Infection and wound dehiscence
   b. Pain or discomfort
2. **Radiographic indications**:
   a. Bone resorption
   b. Loose plates and/or screws, fractured plate
3. **Theoretical indications**:
   a. Stress shielding – Cawood (1985) recommends removal after 3 months for miniplates. For larger fracture plates 6 months is recommended time interval for removal

RIF techniques

There are two opposing schools of thought with regard to RIF of mandible. Some advocate the adaptational monocortical screw fixation whilst others strongly advocate the larger bicortical screw fixation with compression as a means of overcoming the functional forces upon the mandible. The use of one or other technique is a matter of training and personal experience. Both systems work equally well although the compression/bicortical method requires greater surgical exposure with possible longer operating time (Figure 5.1).

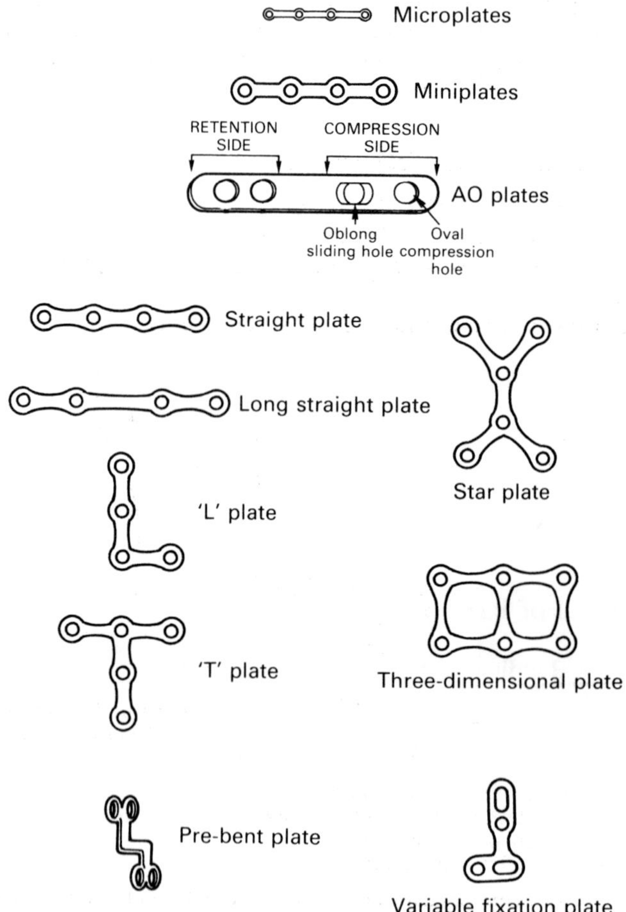

Figure 5.1 Plate sizes and plate shapes.

A. **Adaptational** – miniplates
Monocortical screws and plates (Champy)
B. **Compression**
I. Bicortical screws and plates (AO/ASIF)
II. Lag screws
C. **Mesh systems**

A. Adaptational plating (Figure 5.2)

Champy *et al.* (1976) devised an experimental model of the mandible which mapped out ideal lines of osteosynthesis. By placing plate at most biomechanically favourable site (along tension bands), plate thickness could be kept to a minimum and yet strong enough to overcome displacing forces. Screws need only engage outer cortex.

Physiological stresses of the mandible

1. Tension forces – alveolar border
2. Compression forces – lower border
3. Torsional forces – intercanine region. Two plates required, either:
   a. Lower border and inferior surface plate, *or*

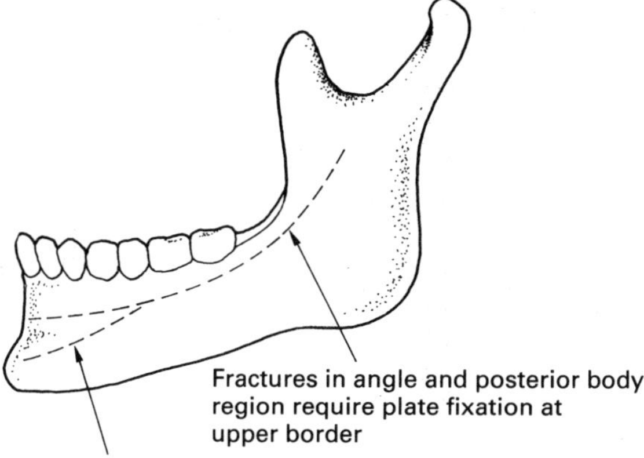

Figure 5.2 Dotted line demonstrates Champy's ideal lines of placement for monocortical plate fixation which follows closely the tension bands created by the forces of the enveloping musculature.

b. Two plates on anterior surface 4–5 mm apart
4. Flexion forces – body of mandible strongest at angle and weakest at premolar region

Adaptational technique of plate fixation

1. Intraoral or transbuccal approach
2. Passive adaptation of plate to bone surface contour
3. Monocortical screw fixation with minimum of two screws on each side of fracture line
4. More posterior fractures require plating at a higher level. More anterior fractures require plating close to the lower border of the mandible
5. To avoid devitalisation of bone the plate should be placed extraperiostally in atrophic edentulous mandibles and also in extensive comminuted fractures

BI. Compression plating

AO – Association of Osteosynthesis
ASIF – Association for the Study of Internal Fixation

First introduced by Spiessl *et al.* in Basel, Switzerland during the early 1970s

AO/ASIF plating system

a. Mandible – used for bridging after resections and for compression of fractures
b. Midface – adaptational miniplates and screws

Compression principles

1. Compression plate (2 mm thick)
   a. Retention side (two holes or more)
   b. Compression side – two or more holes, an oblong sliding hole and an oval compression hole
2. Bicortical pre-tapped screws (2.7 mm diameter)
3. Technique:
   a. Tighten retention screws on one side of fracture
   b. Tighten compression screw on other side of fracture
   c. Tighten screw in sliding hole on same side of fracture as compression screw

4. Limitations – Compression can cause significant occlusal and lingual cortex separation and thus have a limited use in dentate jaws

BII. Lag screw fixation (Figure 5.3)

Describes a **type** of screw as well as a **technique** of screw placement. First used by Brons and Boering (1970) who advised that at least two screws are required to prevent rotational movement of fragments.

Lag screw

Threads are confined to one half of the shaft only, the half nearest the head being smooth. In this way threads engage far cortex of bone while head seats against proximal cortex providing compression of cortices upon tightening

Lag screw technique

Compression is achieved with a normal screw which has threads along its entire length. The hole in the near cortex is enlarged so that threads do not engage.

Techniques
1. Fracture reduced and held in position
2. Hole is drilled through both cortices and hole through near cortex is enlarged

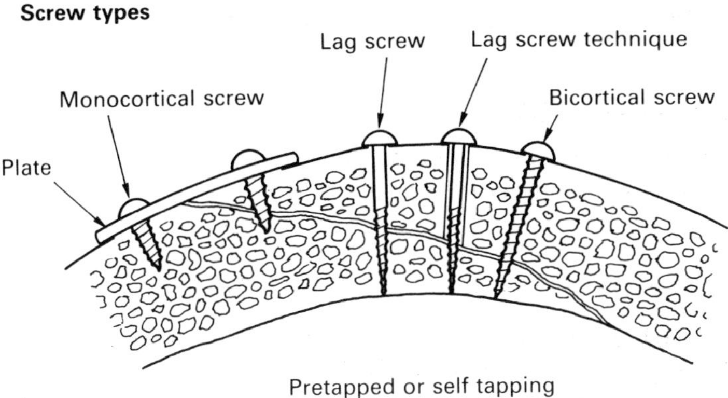

Figure 5.3 Screw and plate techniques for fixing bone fracture of face.

3. Screw is passed into hole and lingual cortex of mandible is engaged and pulled towards buccal cortex for compression
4. Ideally three lag screws should be placed to prevent rotation

Indications

1. Oblique fractures of angle and body of mandible
2. Linear fractures of anterior mandible

Contraindications

Comminuted fractures and areas of bone loss.

Advantages

1. Rapid technique
2. Better anatomical reduction (not proven)
3. Greater rigidity because of compression
4. Cheaper than plates

C. Mesh systems

Alloplastic semi-rigid fixation devices constructed in a mesh pattern to provide a large surface area. This permits adequate rigidity with a reduced thickness and thus a greater degree of adaptability. Useful in complex three-dimensional reconstructions of bony defects.

Functions

1. Provides three-dimensional stability and adaptability
2. Coverage and preservation of bone defects
3. Provides contour and also supports particulate bone grafts

Indications

1. Large bone defects – skull vault, mandibular discontinuity
2. Bone graft support
3. As for other RIF techniques, i.e. airway maintenance and early function

Types

1. Strips
2. Sheets
3. Trays
   a. Segment of mandible
   b. Hemimandible ± condylar prosthesis
   c. Whole mandible ± condylar prostheses

Unique features

Semi-rigid fixation which may:

1. Prevent stress shielding
2. Allow small movements and improve bone healing

Materials for osteosynthesis

1. **Stainless steel**
2. **Cobalt-chrome (Vitallium)**
3. **Titanium**
4. **Bioabsorbable (PLLA – poly-L-lactic acid)**

Stainless steel

Regarded as inferior material with an increased incidence of plate removal

Cobalt-chrome (Vitallium)

Particularly used for microplates

Titanium

1. Pure metal, well tolerated in tissues
2. Chemically inert – corrosion resistant in air and tissue because of titanium oxide layer
3. Low modulus of elasticity – easily deformable and will not spring back after adaptation
4. Non-allergenic
5. Non-magnetic and lightweight
6. Does not interfere with imaging, i.e. CT scans and MRI

Note: Titanium in plates is processed with lower elasticity and hardness than the screws for better deformability

Bio-absorbable materials

Aim: Must be biocompatible with appropriate load-bearing properties and a sufficient rate of degradation that obviates need for removal. As yet there is no reliable material.

Poly-L-lactic acid (PLLA)

Screws and plates with high molecular weight. Microporous and has excellent resilience, although tensile strength is inferior to metallic plates.

1. Biocompatible with little tissue reaction in the short term
2. Rapid decrease of molecular weight and tensile strength over 6 weeks
3. Absorbed by hydrolysis which is estimated to take 3 years
4. Has been used with success in fractured mandibles in dogs and fractured malars in humans
5. Long-term studies have shown foreign body giant cell reaction to PLLA material in tissues over a long period of time

New systems

1. **Microplates** – made of Vitallium or titanium, easily adaptable, used with screws as little as 2 mm long, ideal for craniofacial surgery in babies and surgery to the calvarium
2. **Low profile plates and screws** – particularly useful when plates may be palpated, e.g. at zygomatico-frontal suture
3. **Three-dimensional plates** – a system of plates constructed in a square configuration
4. **Micro-variable plates** – permits adjustment of bone fragments in one or two planes
5. **AO/ASIF–THORP, 3-D** (**T**itanium **HO**llow **R**econstruction **P**lates) – large plates designed to allow minimal contact of hardware with bone graft in order to permit revascularisation of bone graft with osseointegrated screws

Further reading

Cawood J.I. (1985). Small plate osteosynthesis of mandibular fractures. *Br. J. Oral Maxillofac. Surg.*, **23**, 77.

Champy M., Lodde J.P., Schmitt R., Jaeger J.H. and Muster D. (1978). Mandibular osteosynthesis by miniature screwed plates via a buccal approach. *J. Maxillofac. Surg.*, **6**, 14.

Kai Tu.H. and Tenbulzen D. (1985). Compression osteosynthesis of mandibular fractures – a retrospective study. *J. Oral Maxillofac. Surg.*, **43**, 585.

Michelet F.X., Deymes J. and Dessus B. (1973). Osteosynthesis with miniaturised screwed plates in maxillo-facial surgery. *J. Maxillofac. Surg.*, **1**, 79.

Patel M.F. and Langdon J.D. (1991). Titanium mesh (TiMesh) osteosynthesis: a fast and adaptable method of semi-rigid fixation. *Br. J. Oral Maxillofac. Surg.*, **29**, 316.

Pogrel M.A. (1986). Compression osteosynthesis in mandibular fractures. *Int. J. Oral Maxillofac. Surg.*, **15**, 521.

Spiessl B. (1989). *Internal Fixation of the Mandible: A Manual of AO/ASIF Principles*. Berlin: Springer-Verlag.

Worthington P. and Champy M. (1987). Monocortical mini-plate osteosynthesis. *Otolaryngol. Clin. North Am.*, **20**, 607.

Chapter 6

Maxillary fractures

Applied surgical anatomy

The middle third of the face

The area between a horizontal line drawn through supraorbital ridges above and the occlusal plane of the upper teeth or the ridge of the alveolar crest (when edentulous) below. Within this area are the following bones:

Maxillae 2	Inferior conchae 2
Zygomas 2	Pterygoid plates of sphenoid 2
Palatine 2	Vomer
Nasal 2	Ethmoid
Lacrimal 2	

Fracture dynamics of the midface

The midface consists of a series of bony struts passing upwards from upper teeth to base of skull. These bony struts will fracture with severe impact and the middle third of the face is sheared off the cranial base and forced downwards and backwards along an inclined plane formed by the frontal and sphenoid bones. The midface bones absorb most of the fracturing force protecting the bones of the skull base. The clinical features of this displacement of midface include:

1. Apparent trismus – because of posterior gagging of occlusion
2. Lengthening of midface
3. Obstructed airway – soft palate resting on posterior dorsum of tongue
4. Anterior open-bite
5. Dishfaced deformity

Severe fractures of the midface are invariably multiple because a large number of bones are involved.

Classification

Le Fort fractures (Figure 6.1)

Clinically this classification is commonly used. **Réné Le Fort (1901)** experimented by applying trauma to cadaveric heads.

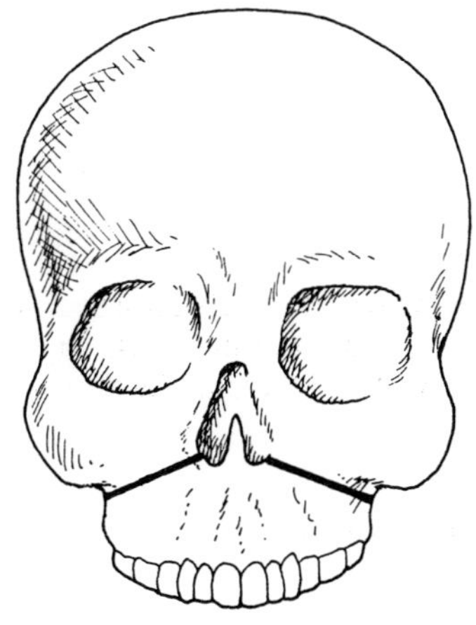

Le Fort I – Low level fracture

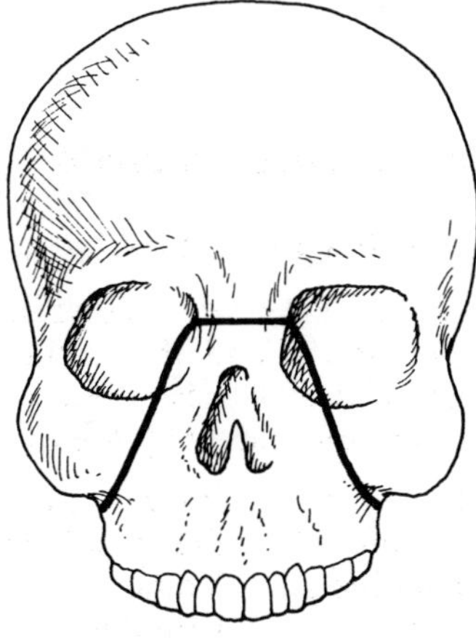

Le Fort II – Pyramidal fracture

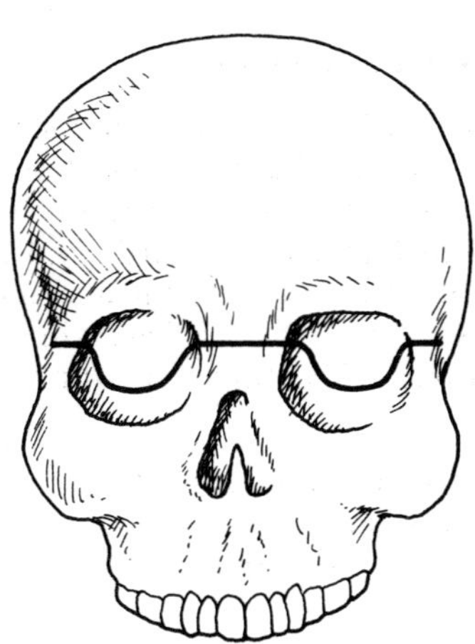

Le Fort III – High level fracture

Figure 6.1 Le Fort type classification for fractures of the middle third of the facial skeleton.

Le Fort I – Guerin or low level fractures
Le Fort II – Pyramidal or subzygomatic fractures
Le Fort III – High level or suprazygomatic fractures

Alternative classification

Middle third facial injuries (Rowe and Williams, 1985)

Fractures not involving the occlusion

1. Central region – key fractures involving:
   a. Nose and/or nasal septum
   b. Fractures of frontal process of maxilla
   c. Naso-ethmoid
   d. Fronto-orbito-nasal
2. Lateral region – zygomatic complex

Fractures involving the occlusion

1. Dento-alveolar fractures
2. Sub-zygomatic:
   Le Fort I
   Le Fort II
3. Supra-zygomatic:
   Le Fort III

Clinical features of midface fractures (Le Fort II,III)

1. Facial swelling – massive oedema
2. Bilateral circumorbital ecchymoses – panda facies, or raccoon eyes
3. Bilateral subconjunctival ecchymosis
4. Lengthening of face
5. Abnormal mobility of midface
6. Pain over nose and face
7. Malocclusion – anterior open-bite
8. Diplopia
9. Anaesthesia – infraorbital nerves damaged
10. Blood and cerebrospinal fluid discharging from the nose

Surgical treatment planning

Timing of surgical procedures

A. Emergency treatment – resuscitate patient

1. Stabilize mobile fractures to maintain airway (need for tracheóstomy?)
2. Arrest haemorrhage and transfuse if necessary
3. Monitor vital signs

B. Within 24 hours

1. Repair deep lacerations
2. Impressions of teeth
3. Treat less-severe maxillary fractures if no other major injuries

C. Definitive treatment (days 2–8)

Optimal time to allow for:

1. Improvement in medical condition of patient
2. Careful clinical assessment and planning
3. Reduction of soft-tissue oedema

Stages of surgical procedure in patient with multiple facial injuries

1. Tracheostomy if required
2. Dento-alveolar fractures:
   a. Extract teeth beyond repair
   b. Reduction and fixation of dento-alveolar fragments
3. Reduction of mandibular fractures – to act as guide for correct positioning of maxilla
4. Zygomatic fractures – should be elevated to allow greater disimpaction of maxillae
5. Disimpaction and reduction of maxillae:
   a. Open
   b. Closed
6. Skeletal fixation:
   a. Internal
      i. Non-rigid
         Suspension wiring
         Intramedullary pins
         Transosseous wiring

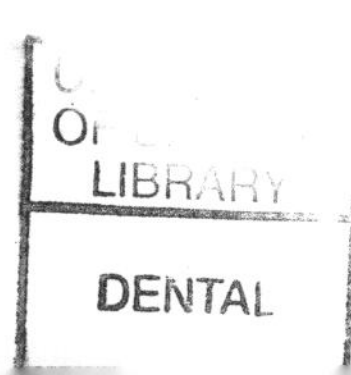

ii. Rigid
Adaptational plates
Monocortical screws
b. External
i. External pin fixation via frame or halo
7. Reduction and fixation of nasal fractures
8. Facial lacerations – give access to fracture sites:
a. Clean and repair
b. Care of facial nerve, lacrimal apparatus, or parotid duct if indicated

Treatment of maxillary fractures (Figure 6.2)

1. **Internal skeletal fixation**
   a. Rigid internal fixation
   b. Wire suspension
   c. Transfixion – K wires
   d. Transosseous wires
2. **External skeletal fixation**
   a. Halo frame
   b. Levant frame
   c. Box frame

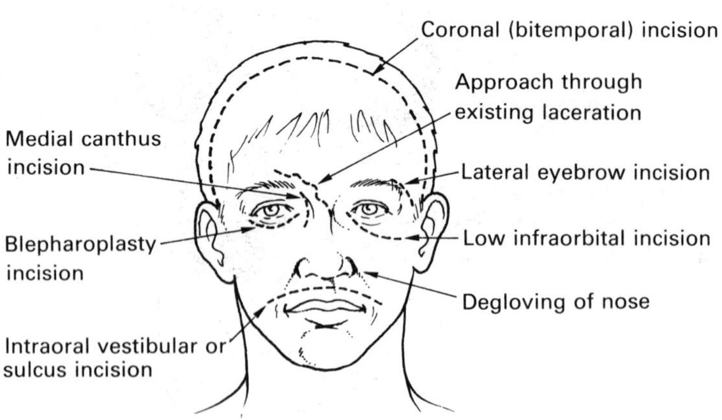

Figure 6.2 Some of the more common incisions for approaches to fractures of the middle third of the face.

Rigid internal fixation (see Chapter 5) (Figure 6.3)

Rigid fixation in the maxillofacial region has only developed in the last decade or two with the advent of miniaturised orthopaedic plates and screws. Operative complications associated with the use of rigid fixation are decreasing with improvement in design of plates and operating techniques.

Champy *et al.* (1977) advise that plating should commence at the periphery – i.e. zygomatico-frontal suture and mandible before proceeding towards plating of the central midface area (i.e. orbital-naso-ethmoidal areas).

Initial plating of frontal process of maxilla to the frontal bone provides rigid vertical anterior support for Le Fort II and III fractures.

Principles of plating midface

Must restore supporting pillars that take up masticatory forces. Miniplates must lie in the longitudinal direction of these pillars.

1. Microplates – orbit, naso-ethmoidal areas

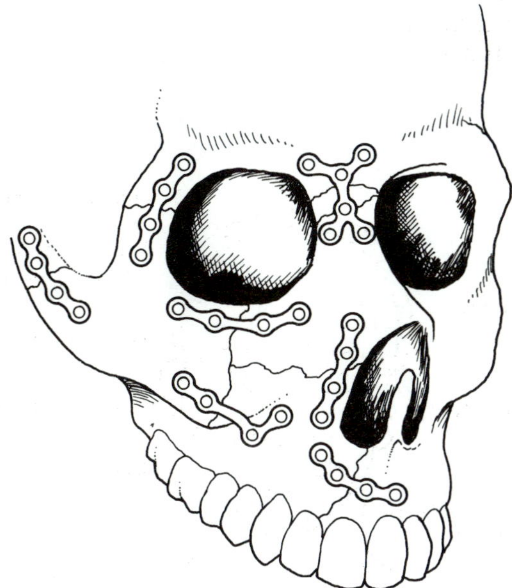

Figure 6.3 Placement of monocortical screws and plate fixation for the treatment of midface fractures.

2. Miniplates – malar and maxillary fractures
3. Compression plates – sometimes used on mandible

Wire suspension (Figure 6.4)

Adams 1942 used to reduce and suspend a mobile fragment below to a firm stable fragment above the fracture by means of a 0.5 mm stainless steel wire.

Advantages

1. Comfortable, well tolerated and inconspicuous
2. Rapid technique, accurate and dependable

Disadvantages

1. Non-rigid fixation
2. The suspension wires may exert a backward and upward pull which may lead to relapse of reduced maxilla
3. Requires intermaxillary fixation

Frontal suspension

Incision lateral third of eyebrow to expose zygomatico-frontal suture. Burr hole drilled above zygomatico-frontal suture and emerges in infratemporal fossa. Using **Rowe's zygomatic awl** both ends of wire passed into mouth through upper buccal sulcus.

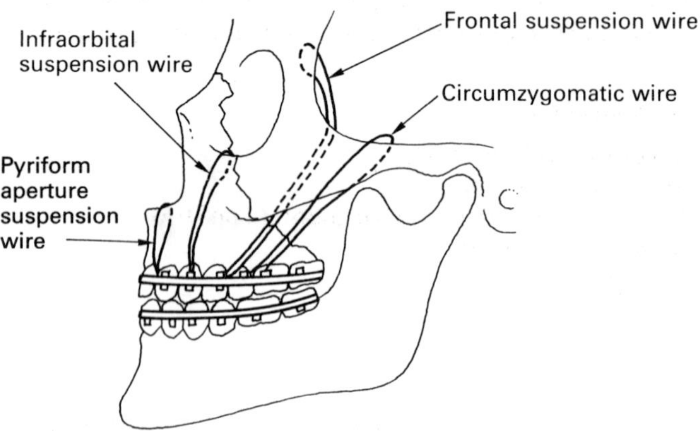

Figure 6.4 Wire suspension of midface fractures.

Circumzygomatic suspension

Circumzygomatic wires passed and attached to arch bars on maxillary teeth.

Zygomatic suspension

Base of zygomatic buttress exposed via buccal sulcus incision and wire inserted through a drilled hole.

Infraorbital suspension

Through upper labial sulcus incision.

Pyriform aperture suspension

Bony pyriform aperture of nose exposed via upper labial sulcus incision and wire passed through.

Circumpalatal wire

Longitudinal wire passed around palate provides good retention for surgical splint following maxillectomy and superior stability of gunning splint to maxilla.

External skeletal fixation (Figure 6.5)

Involves the use of external rods and universal joints which link the cranium above the fracture to maxilla or mandible via an extension rod wired rigidly to the teeth. Used to provide anterior traction to the midface which is unstable antero-posteriorly.

Contraindications

1. Severe scalp lacerations
2. Skull fractures
3. Heavy cerebral irritation or mental confusion
4. Mentally deranged
5. Epilepsy
6. Alcoholism

Halo frame

Partially or completely encircles head but difficult to sleep with, e.g. Royal Berkshire Hospital pattern

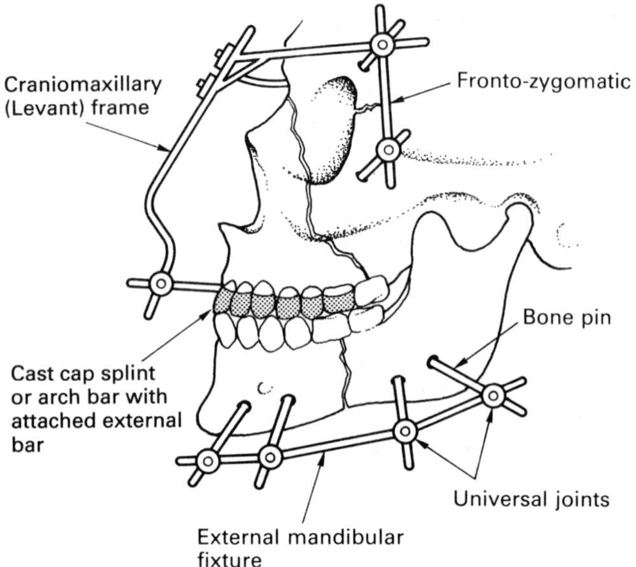

Figure 6.5 External pin fixation for maxillofacial fractures.

Levant frame

Developed at Royal Melbourne Hospital 1960s. Craniomaxillary fixation between supraorbital ridges and maxilla.

Advantages
1. Rigid, light with minimal bulk
2. Simple design and application, rapidly applied
3. Does not interfere with urgent neurosurgical procedures or vision
4. Can maintain position of maxilla in absence of IMF

Construction
1. Bilateral 30 degree bends of horizontal arm
2. Supraorbital Toller or Moule pins and universal joints for cranial fixation
3. Central vertical rod attached by means of two universal joints

Box frame

Craniomandibular fixation; middle third of face is sandwiched between mandible and cranium. Difficult to release jaws in emergency.

Complications of major maxillary fractures

Preoperative complications

1. Airway – posteriorly displaced maxilla causes soft palate to rest on dorsal surface of tongue
2. Bleeding – severe epistaxis related to bleeding from maxillary arteries
3. Inhalation – tooth fragments

Postoperative complications

1. Excessive bleeding – may need transfusion
2. Infection – wound dehiscence
   emphysema
   meningitis (CSF leak) very rare
3. Malocclusion
4. Facial scarring
5. Non-vital teeth

Rehabilitation

- Facial scar revision
- Dental rehabilitation
- Post-traumatic facial deformity correction
- Social and psychiatric report

Further reading

Adams W.M. and Adams L.H. (1956). Internal wire fixation of facial fractures: a fifteen year follow-up report. *Am. J. Surg.*, **92**, 12.

Banks P. (1987). *Killey's Fractures of the Middle Third of the Facial Skeleton* 5th edn. Oxford: Butterworth-Heinemann (Wright).

Bowerman J.E. (1985). *Maxillofacial Injuries* vol. 1, (Rowe N.L. and Williams J.Ll., eds). Edinburgh: Churchill Livingstone, chap. 11.

Le Fort R. (1901). Experimental studies of fractures of the upper jaw (translated from the French by Tessier P). *Plast. Reconstr. Surg.*, **50**, 600.

Steidler N., Cook R.M. and Reade P.C. (1980). Residual complications in patients with major middle third facial fractures. *Int. J. Oral Surg.*, **9**, 259.

Chapter 7

Zygomatic fractures

Applied surgical anatomy

Functions of zygoma

1. Protection of globe of eye
2. To give origin to masseter muscle – zygomatic arch
3. To transmit part of masticatory forces to cranial base

Axis of rotation for fractures (Figure 7.1)

1. Vertical plane – Fronto-zygomatic (F–Z) suture, zygomatic bone and buttress, first molar tooth
2. Horizontal plane – inferior orbital margin and zygomatic arch

Classification of zygomatic fractures (Henderson, 1973)

Type 1 – Undisplaced fracture
Type 2 – Arch fracture only

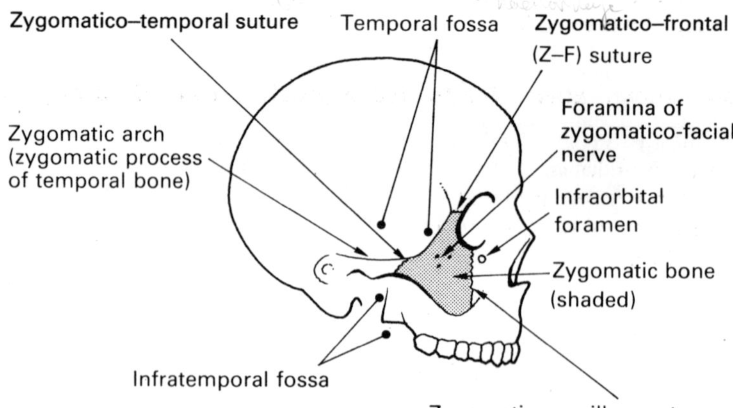

Figure 7.1 The zygomatic bone in relation to the rest of the facial skeleton.

Type 3 – Tripod malar fracture (F–Z suture intact)
Type 4 – Tripod malar fracture (F–Z suture distracted)
Type 5 – Pure blowout fracture
Type 6 – Orbital rim fracture
Type 7 – Comminuted and other fractures

Clinical features

Early

1. Swelling and bruising over cheek
2. Depressed cheek prominence
3. Trismus and restricted lateral mandibular movements
4. Step deformity along infraorbital margin and possibly along lateral orbital margin and zygomatic buttress
5. Diplopia
6. Sometimes exophthalmos
7. Periorbital ecchymosis and subconjunctival haemorrhage. A subconjunctival haemorrhage has no posterior limit. The blood remains bright red for a number of weeks because of diffusion of oxygen across the conjunctiva
8. Anaesthesia or paraesthesia of infraorbital and anterior superior alveolar nerve. If full recovery occurs it may take 5–9 months. Proximal part of nerve recovers first, i.e. cheek before upper lip. After 1 year 10% still complain of paraesthesia.
9. Paraesthesia or anaesthesia of zygomatico-facial and zygomatico-temporal nerves. This gives anaesthesia of prominence of cheek and temple respectively
10. Epistaxis on side of fracture

Late – complications of untreated or poorly treated fractures

1. Flat cheek
2. Enophthalmos
3. Altered pupillary level
4. Infraorbital paraesthesia
5. Diplopia

Radiographs

Occipitomental 15 and 30 degrees

- Step in infraorbital margin
- Separation of F–Z suture

- Fracture of zygomatic arch and buttress
- Opaque maxillary sinus

Submentovertical

- Fracture of zygomatic arch

Historical review

Ferrier 1825 – attempted to reduce a fractured malar through an incision above the arch
Stroymeyer 1844 – was the first to suggest elevating a malar using a percutaneous hook
Dupuytren 1847 – identified the importance of the plane between temporal fascia and the temporal muscle
Cheyne *et al*. 1901 – suggested the use of intraoral digital manipulation of a fractured malar
Gillies *et al*. 1927 – described the temporal incision within hairline as of cosmetic value

Non-surgical management

Reserved for the following cases:

1. Medical contraindications
2. Very elderly
3. Minimal displacement

Rowe and Killey 1970 – in a series of over 300 zygomatic fractures nearly 20% did not require treatment

Surgical intervention

Indications

1. Flat cheek
2. Diplopia
3. Infraorbital paraesthesia – not certain that surgery improves recovery
4. Impaired mandibular movement

Time

As soon as possible – elevation becomes difficult after 14 days. Delay allows:

1. Dispersion of gross oedema
2. Proper ophthalmic examination. A zygomatic fracture will be firmly united in 3–4 weeks

Other considerations when deciding urgency of surgery

1. Progressive deterioration of vision as in retrobulbar haemorrhage – very urgent surgery.
2. The necessity for immediate surgery because of other injuries.
3. Medical condition of patient.

Surgical approaches to the zygoma

1. **Temporal fossa**
2. **Intraoral**
3. **Percutaneous** – stab incision for hook, eyebrow incision, bicoronal flap

Temporal fossa approach (Gillies *et al.*, 1927)

1. Oblique 45 degree incision made in hairline, parallel to anterior branch of superficial temporal artery above bifurcation
2. Temporal fascia exposed and incised
3. Howarth elevator passed below zygoma between temporalis fascia and temporalis muscle; this acts as a guide for introduction of an elevator, e.g. Rowe's zygomatic elevator
4. Firm upward and outward elevation is applied
5. Postoperatively pressure on fractured malar should be avoided allowing healing within 3 weeks
   For direct access to malar a preauricular incision (Al-Kayat and Bramley, 1979) is used.

Intraoral approach

Access via 1 cm incision in upper buccal sulcus immediately behind the zygomatic buttress, pointed curved elevator (Taylor–Monk's pattern) passed upwards to contact intratemporal surface of zygoma allowing elevation of malar.

Percutaneous approach

1. Stab incision placed at intersection of:
   a. Vertical line dropped from outer canthus of eye
   b. Horizontal line extending from alar margin of nostril

   Poswillo hook is inserted through incision below and behind the malar prominence. Reduction is achieved by strong outward traction of the handle avoiding infraorbital fissure which may result in haemorrhage from vein traversing it
2. Eyebrow incision allows elevation of malar together with placing of a plate across zygomatico-frontal suture
3. Bicoronal flap – can be used when flap is raised for other reasons, e.g. exploration of anterior cranial fossa

Stability of zygomatic fractures

Stability of fracture depends on

1. Attachment of temporalis fascia superiorly which counteracts displacing effect of masseter muscle inferiorly
2. Adequacy and accuracy of bony apposition at fracture sites – the periosteum should be kept as intact as possible, this means a fractured zygoma should not be overelevated or it will tear periosteum.

Fractures which may require fixation

1. Separation of F–Z suture and disruption of infraorbital margin
2. Comminuted fractures
3. Arch fracture
4. Delayed treatment leading to fibrosis and resorption of fracture lines

Methods of stabilisation

1. Osteosynthesis
   a. Direct wiring
   b. Miniplates or microplates
2. Antral support
   a. Antral pack
   b. Balloon
   c. Silicone wedge used to underpin zygomatic buttress and removed 6 months later

3. External pin fixation
   F–Z
4. Internal pin fixation
   a. Transmaxillary K-wire
   b. Naso-maxillary K-wire

Osteosynthesis

- Transosseous wires may not be sufficient to rigidly fix F–Z suture
- Plates supply best stability and are commonly used (Figure 7.2)

Antral support

- Used as a supplementary measure when there is gross comminution of the zygoma, with or without an intact orbital floor
- Antral pack usually gauze soaked in Whitehead's varnish
- Balloon applies unfavourable forces and is seldom used

External pin fixation

- F–Z – pin placed in body of zygoma rigidly fixed to supra-orbital pin with vertical rod

Internal pin fixation

1. Transmaxillary – opposite unfractured zygoma used to rigidly hold fractured zygoma in place using K-wire. This K-wire is passed transversely through intact zygoma across face into

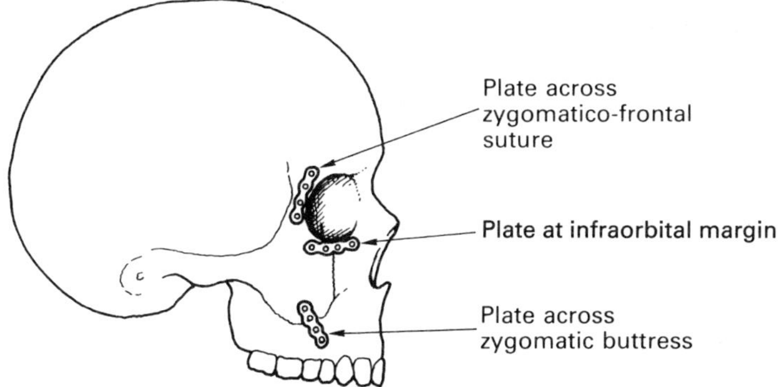

Figure 7.2 Stabilization of fractured zygoma with plates.

fractured malar. Beware accidentally transfixing eyeball or nasal anaesthetic tube. Pin removal at 3–6 weeks
2. Naso-zygomatic – transnasal K-wire inserted from frontal process of maxilla to contralateral fractured zygoma

Further reading

Al-Kayat A. and Bramley P. (1979). A modified pre-auricular approach to the temporomandibular joint and malar arch. *Br. J. Oral Surg.*, **17**, 91.

Balasubramanian S. (1967). Intra-oral approach for reduction of malar fractures. *Br. J. Oral Surg.*, **4**, 189.

Banks P. (1987). *Killey's Fractures of the Middle Third of the Facial Skeleton*, 5th edn. Oxford: Butterworth-Heinemann (Wright).

Ellis E. (1991). Fractures of the zygomatic complex and arch. In Oral and Maxillofacial Trauma vol. 1 (Fonseca R.J. and Walker R.V., eds). Philadelphia: W.B. Saunder, chap. 18.

Finlay P.M., Ward-Booth R.P. and Moos K.F. (1984). Morbidity associated with the use of antral packs and external pins in the treatment of the unstable fracture of the zygomatic complex. *Br. J. Oral Surg.*, **22**, 18.

Gillies H.D., Kilner T.P. and Stone D. (1927). Fractures of the malar–zygomatic compound, with a description of a new X-ray position. *Br. J. Surg.*, **14**, 651.

Rowe N.L. and Williams J.Ll., eds (1985). *Maxillofacial Injuries* vol. 1 Edinburgh: Churchill Livingstone, chap. 12.

Chapter 8

Orbital injuries

Surgical anatomy (Figure 8.1)

Fractures of the orbital rim

Fractures caused by a localised severe blow – such a fracture can extend to involve associated orbital wall.

Anatomical structures related to:

1. Inferior rim include – infraorbital nerve
   inferior oblique muscle

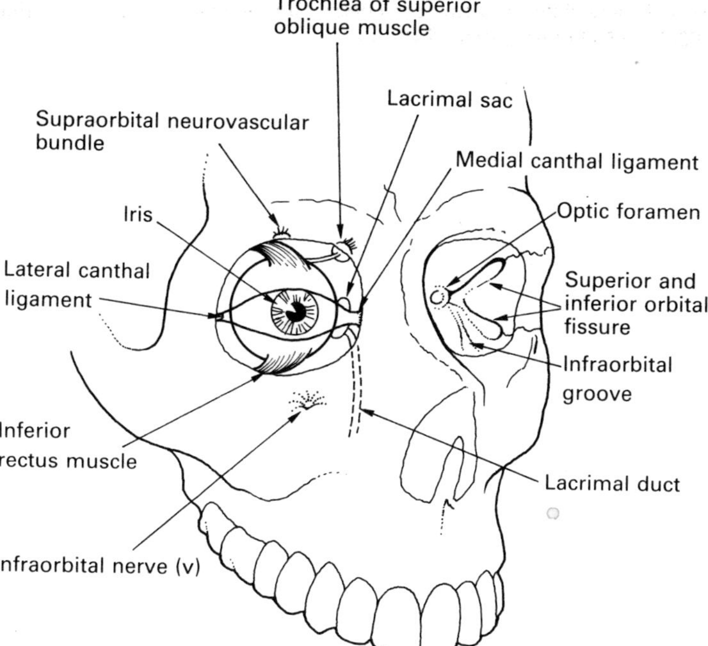

Figure 8.1 Important surgical landmarks which may be disrupted by orbital fractures.

2. Superior rim include – lacrimal gland
   supraorbital nerve
   frontal sinus
3. Lateral rim – lateral canthal ligament
4. Medial rim – medial canthal ligament
   lacrimal apparatus

Fractures of the orbital walls

Fractures of roof and lateral wall of the orbit tend to involve the orbital rim. Isolated fractures tend to involve orbital floor and medial wall (blowout). An orbital floor fracture may involve infraorbital nerve, inferior rectus and inferior oblique muscles. A medial wall fracture may involve the lacrimal apparatus, medial rectus and suspensory ligament.

Clinical features

Numerous signs and symptoms can be related to orbital injuries. The signs and symptoms are related to type and site of injury. Examination by an ophthalmologist may not alter the type of orbital fracture repair but may well influence the indications and timing for such a repair.

Early signs and symptoms

1. **The periorbital tissues**:
   a. Oedema
   b. Ecchymosis
   c. Surgical emphysema
      i. Related to injury, usually a crack fracture between orbit and paranasal sinus
      ii. Crackling sensation on palpation usually after blowing nose
      iii. Air with nasal pathogens may cause an infection such as orbital cellulitis requiring antibiotics. Recovers spontaneously in a few days
2. **Eyelids**:
   a. Lacerations of the eyelids
   b. Ptosis – drooping of the eyelid which can be caused by haemorrhage, oedema or neurological damage

3. **Eye**:
   a. Oculomotor (III) nerve injury
   b. Proptosis – protrusion of eyeball caused by
      i. Oedema
      ii. Bleeding – particularly a retrobulbar haemorrhage (see below)
   c. Telecanthus = increased intercanthal distance > 35 mm due to avulsion of the medial canthal ligaments (normal intercanthal distance 25–35 mm)
      (Hypertelorism = increased interpupillary distance)
   d. Subconjunctival haemorrhage
   e. Loss of visual acuity
   f. Loss of pupillary reflexes
      i. Loss of pupil light reflex in injured eye indicates damage to the optic nerve or damage to oculomotor nerve
      ii. Loss of consensual reflex in injured eye indicates injury to oculomotor nerve
   g. Traumatic mydriasis (dilatation of pupil)
   h. Traumatic miosis (constriction of pupil)
   i. Diplopia
      i. Oedema
      ii. Muscle trapping
      iii. Paresis of extraocular muscles
   j. Lacrimal apparatus – wounds involving the puncta, lacrimal canaliculi or nasolacrimal duct may damage or obstruct them causing epiphora
4. **Neurological defects** – paraesthesia or anaesthesia of supraorbital or supratrochlear nerve (Va) or infraorbital nerve (Vb)
5. **Paralysis** – of the extraocular muscles related to oculomotor (III) trochlear (IV) or abducent (VI) nerve injuries
6. **Bony orbital rim** – visible deformity or palpable deformity and pain
7. **CSF leak** – related to fracture of medial orbital wall and cribiform plate. May cause fluctuant swelling in upper medial aspect of supratarsal fold; may cause CSF rhinorrhoea

Late signs and symptoms

Usually concealed by bruising and swelling in the acute phase. These features occur between a few days and several weeks after injury. They may be related to untreated or poorly treated injuries. Many of the early signs and symptoms may persist, e.g. nerve paraesthesias or paralysis.

1. **Eyelids**:
   a. Changes in palpebral fissure – Mongoloid or antimongoloid slant due to damage sustained to medial and lateral canthal ligaments (usually avulsion)
   b. With moderate enophthalmos the palpebral fissure may be widened giving appearance of a staring eye
   c. In severe enophthalmos the palpebral fissure is usually narrowed
2. **Eye**:
   a. Enophthalmos
      i. Posterior recession of the globe (see blowout fractures). Usually the eye sinks in 1–4 mm
   b. Drop in ocular level (hypoglobus)
      i. Directly related to avulsion of suspensory ligament
      ii. Indirectly related to bony displacement, e.g. separation of F–Z suture

Blowout fractures (Figure 8.2)

Fracture of the orbital floor with an intact orbital rim. They can affect orbital floor or medial orbital wall.

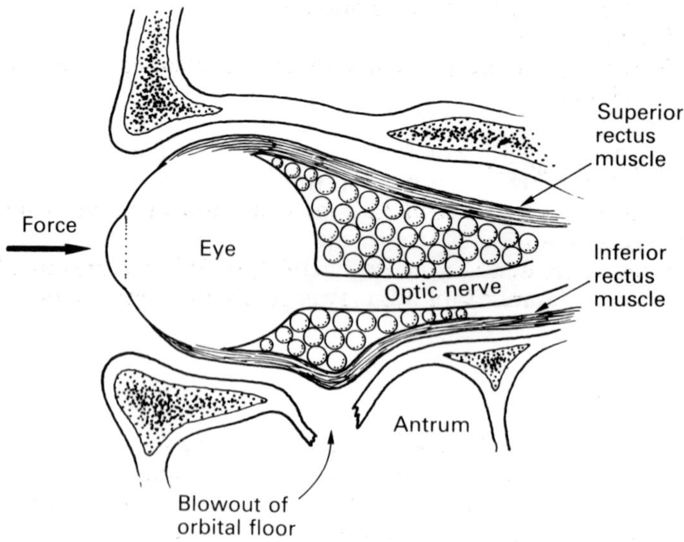

Figure 8.2 Mechanism of blowout fracture.

Aetiology

Isolated orbital floor fracture (pure blowout):

- Blunt trauma to eye whereby kinetic energy is transmitted to surrounding fat and thence to orbital walls
- Most common cause is punch in eye

May form part of more extensive fracture:

- Zygoma
- Extension of orbital rim fracture
- Le Fort II and III midface fractures

Clinical features

Early signs and symptoms

1. Periorbital oedema and ecchymosis
2. Limited upward rotation of eye with pain
3. Paraesthesia of infraorbital nerve
4. Proptosis and diplopia

Late signs and symptoms (10 days or more)

1. Restricted vertical eye movements with pain
2. Diplopia
3. Altered ocular level (hypoglobus)
4. Enophthalmos
5. Narrowing of the palpebral fissure, deepening of the supratarsal fold

Optic nerve trauma

Caused indirectly by stretching or contusion of nerve – skeletal fractures.

In the series of Crumley *et al*. (1977) of 363 fractures involving the orbital floor, there was damage to the optic nerve in 28 (7.7%).

Radiographs

1. **Occipitomental 15 and 30 degrees** – hanging drop opacity in roof of antrum. Fracture of zygoma or maxilla
2. **CT scan** – coronal scan easily identifies blowout fracture
3. **Orbital tomography** – shows hanging drop opacity in roof of antrum. Rarely used because of large dose of radiation

Investigations

Forced duction test

Tendon of inferior rectus muscle grasped by forceps through the conjunctiva and eye is rotated upwards, resistance to free movement indicates that there is mechanical trapping

- Herniation of orbital fat
- Entrapment of muscle
- Adhesions

A negative forced duction test in early post-traumatic period does not exclude possibility of herniation of tissues into the antrum since fibrous tissue will not have formed until 10 days later.
This test can be equivocal.

Retraction test

Posterior movement of globe when antagonist muscle is unable to 'pay out rope' so that axis of rotation is transferred to site of restriction or adhesion.

Treatment of orbital floor fractures

Indications for surgical intervention

1. Positive forced duction test
2. Diplopia – particularly on looking upwards
3. Restricted eye movements – particularly when looking upwards
4. Pain when moving eye
5. When CT scan reveals blowout fracture

Preoperative considerations

1. Check visual acuity prior to surgery
2. Consider waiting until swelling has subsided

Surgical objectives

1. Repositioning of displaced orbital tissues
2. Restoration of orbital floor

3. Reduction and stabilisation of causative fractures
4. Free movement of globe

Surgical procedures

1. **Orbital floor grafting** – the majority of cases
2. **Antral support** – when orbital floor fragments are sagging into antrum, useful when there is an associated comminuted fracture of zygoma
3. **Combined** – antral pack to support graft, may increase risk of infection

Surgical approach to orbital floor (Figure 8.3)

A. Transconjunctival incision

Incision is made on inner aspect of lower eyelid. The advantage is an invisible scar. The disadvantages are:

- Limited access to orbital floor
- Significant risk of herniating fat of lower eyelid (originally developed by Bourguet 1928 as a cosmetic procedure for fat herniation of lower eyelid)

B. Infraorbital incision

1. **Blepharoplasty (subciliary)** – Incision made parallel to lower margin of eyelid, usually in skin crease 2 mm below lid margin: provides excellent exposure of entire orbital floor and

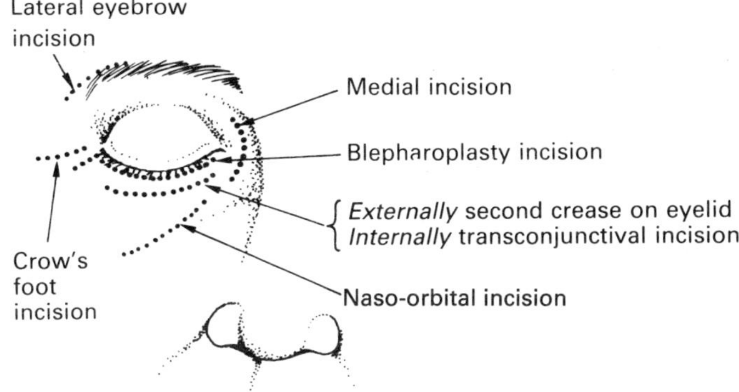

Figure 8.3 Surgical approaches to orbit.

lower part of lateral and medial walls of orbit. Incision can be extended in crow's foot to increase exposure of orbital floor and zygoma. Step incisions at different levels:

- Skin
- Orbicularis oculi muscle
- Periosteum

Complications include ectropion – eversion of lower eyelid

2. **Second crease of lower eyelid** – good surgical exposure
3. **Naso-orbital incision** – Provides good access to medial orbital floor; heals very well when orbit is oedematous or bruised

Orbital floor grafts

Functions of an orbital floor graft

1. Repair of orbital floor
2. Inert surface which will not form adhesions
3. Restore contour and volume of orbit
4. Support to globe

Ideal implants

1. Biocompatible, non-allergenic and non-carcinogenic materials which can be sterilised
2. Strong, rigid and adaptable to sculpting at operation
3. Easy to anchor into position
4. Should unite to surrounding bone or become encapsulated by fibrous tissue

Autografts

These are grafts of the patient's own tissues to the orbital floor

Donor sites

1. Antral wall – where Caldwell–Luc approach is employed
2. Nasal septal cartilage
3. Outer table of bone from calvarium
4. Inner plate of iliac crest – where curvature corresponds closely to curvature of orbital floor
5. Split rib – cortex forming orbital floor
6. Cartilage – rib or pinna of ear

Indications

Particularly useful in large orbital floor defects and malunited fractures.

Special considerations

Cortical surface of bone must face orbit – about 25% of bone graft will resorb. Cartilage has a better prognosis than bone because it has a lower rate of metabolism and survives well under relatively anaerobic conditions.

Autografts also have the disadvantage of

1. Additional surgery to harvest graft
2. Correct placement can be difficult to achieve

Allografts

1. **Processed bovine bone** – framework is eventually replaced by living bone from host
2. **Lyophilised dura mater** – now rarely used because of risk of Creutzfeldt–Jakob disease caused by a slow virus
3. **Zenoderm** – porcine skin

Alloplastic grafts

Inert foreign body which becomes encapsulated by fibrous tissue but does not undergo any physical change. Implants lie passively in place after being inserted in subperiosteal plane.

Dacron reinforced silastic

Dimethyl siloxane polymer. Thin sheet (0.4 mm) of flexible material, cut to shape and secured to rim with wires, stainless steel sutures, or butyl cyanoacrylate glue.

Antral packing

Indications

1. Small orbital floor defect
2. Comminuted fractures of orbital floor still attached to periosteum

3. Where prolapsed antral soft tissues can be replaced in orbit
4. No adhesions restricting ocular mobility

Limitations

1. Infection
2. Poor control of orbital floor

Approach to antrum

Caldwell–Luc.
Incision in upper buccal sulcus in canine fossa region. Window made in bony lateral wall of antrum

Antral pack

1. Ribbon gauze – half-inch soaked in Whitehead's varnish (pigmented Iodoform compound)
2. Approximate capacity of antrum = 30 ml
3. Contents of Whitehead's varnish = Iodoform 10 g, Benzoin 10 g, Storax 7.5 g, Tolubalsam 5 g, Solvent Ether to 100 ml.
4. End of pack can be left protruding through incision in upper buccal sulcus **or** end of pack can be sealed into antrum
5. Pack remains in place for approximately 3 weeks
6. Easily removed via incision in buccal sulcus under LA
7. Pack should:
   a. Exert passive force
   b. Prevent infection

Antral balloon

1. Foley catheter inserted into antrum and end of tubing led out through nostril
2. Sterile saline is slowly injected to fill catheter until required degree of reduction is achieved. Radiopaque solution may be used
3. Removed after approximately 14 days
4. Correct supporting pressure is not achieved to the same extent as a Whitehead's varnish pack – rarely used

Postoperative considerations

1. Ophthalmoscopic examination of globe
2. Pupil reflexes

3. Antibiotic drops – chloramphenicol 0.5% or 1%
4. Eye and periorbital tissues left uncovered to avoid direct pressure
5. Sutures removed about 5 days after surgery
6. Firm clinical union in 3 weeks in case of associated fracture

Complications of orbital fractures

Retrobulbar haemorrhage

Rare complication resulting from orbital trauma or surgical intervention (in 1000 malar fractures in the series of Ord (1981), 0.3% developed retrobulbar haemorrhage postoperatively).

Mechanism

1. **Bleeding behind the eye** – Sometimes divided into extraconal and intraconal bleeding. The 'cone' being the cone of extraocular muscle. Bleeding inside this cone occurs from ciliary arteries and may cause venous congestion and oedema around anterior head of optic nerve. Known as anterior ischaemic optic neuropathy (AION) and causes blindness
2. Sometimes a retrobulbar haemorrhage may cause compression of central retinal artery causing blindness

Signs and symptoms

- Deteriorating vision or blindness
- Ophthalmoplegia
- Proptosis
- Tense globe
- Marked chemosis and ecchymosis
- Dilated pupil
- Loss of direct pupil reflex
- Retention of consensual light reflex
- Pain in the eye

Treatment

Untreated there is irreversible ischaemia of retinal cells and permanent blindness

Medical
Aimed at decreasing intraocular pressure:

1. Acetazolamide (Diamox) 500 mg i.v.
2. Large doses of i.v. steroids (dexamethasone 3–4 mg/kg)
3. Dehydration with mannitol 200 ml in 20% solution i.v.
4. Papaverine 40 mg i.v.

Surgery
Decompression of orbit:

1. Infraorbital incision and blunt dissection into intraconal space
2. Lateral canthotomy.

Orbit should always be drained but medical treatment can be given until patient can be operated upon. Measurement with exophthalmometer at surgery indicates decompression of orbit

Superior orbital fissure syndrome (Figure 8.4)

Rare damage to structures which pass through superior orbital fissure.

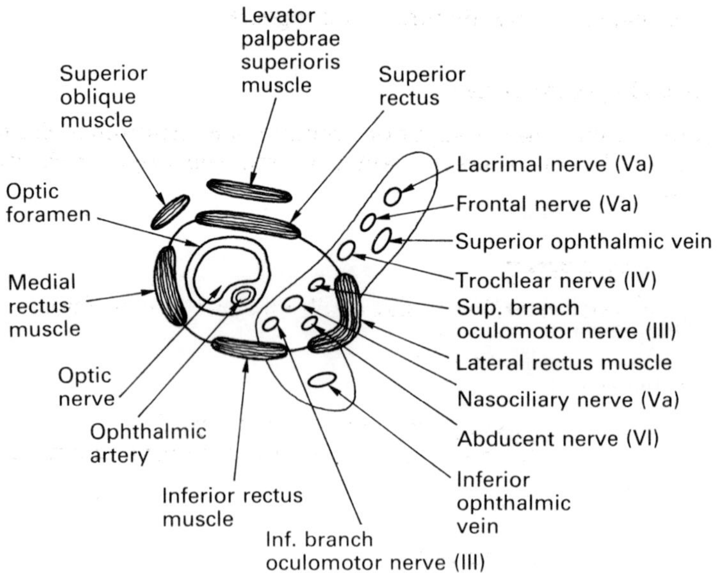

Figure 8.4 Left superior orbital fissure and tendinous ring of origin of extraocular muscles.

Nerves

Superior and inferior branches of III, IV, Va (frontal nasociliary and lacrimal), VI together with ophthalmic veins.

Signs and symptoms

- Proptosis and subconjunctival haemorrhage
- Oedema of the periorbita
- Dilated pupil
- Light reflex absent
- Consensual reflex present
- Loss of accommodation of eye
- Sensory loss of cornea and forehead

Imaging

Radiographic or CT scan evidence of reduction in size of superior orbital fissure.

Treatment

1. Wait and see policy
2. Great care if treating fractured zygoma

Orbital apex syndrome

Rare combination of superior orbital fissure syndrome with damage to the optic nerve. Anterior ischaemic optic neuropathy (AION).

Signs and symptoms

As for superior orbital fissure syndrome with loss of vision

Treatment

1. Usually no treatment indicated if eye is blind
2. Progressive loss of vision may indicate surgical decompression of optic canal

Carotico-cavernous fistula

Rare orbital injury leading to carotid artery tear within cavernous sinus

Signs and symptoms

- Pulsating exophthalmos
- Subconjunctival haemorrhage
- Ophthalmoplegia
- Dilated pupil
- Reduced vision

Treatment

Surgical closure of fistula or embolisation

Traumatic enophthalmos

Definition

Posterior recession of the globe following trauma. This is a late complication.

Causes

1. Outward displacement of orbital floor or medial orbital wall, i.e. blowout fracture
2. Loss of periorbital fat volume:
   a. Herniation of fat into maxillary sinus or other cavities
   b. Fat fibrosis and atrophy

Signs and Symptoms

1. Pseudo-ptosis – deepening of supratarsal crease leading to narrowing of palpebral fissure
2. Diplopia
3. Usually infraorbital paraesthesia

Treatment

This should be aimed at anticipating and preventing the development of enophthalmos. If enophthalmos develops early treatment will minimise it. The repair of late post-traumatic enophthalmos is usually not a very successful procedure. The prevention of enophthalmos involves early treatment of orbital floor fractures (see above).

Further reading

Banks P. (1987). *Killey's Fractures of the Middle Third of the Facial Skeleton*, 5th edn. Oxford: Butterworth-Heinemann (Wright).

Banks P. (1967). The superior orbital fissure syndrome. *Oral Surg. Oral Med. Oral Pathol.*, **24**, 455.

Barber H.D. and Betts N.J. (1993). The biomechanics of orbitozygomatic fractures and concepts of rigid internal fixation. *Oral Maxillofac. Surg. Clin. North Am.*, **5**, 457.

Converse J.M. and Smith B. (1957). Enophthalmos and diplopia in fractures of the orbital floor. *Br. J. Plast. Surg.*, **9**, 265.

Crikelair G.F., *et al*. (1972). A critical look at the 'blowout' fracture. *Plast. Reconstr. Surg.*, **49**, 374.

Fujino T. (1974). Experimental blowout fracture of the orbit. *Plast. Reconstr. Surg.*, **54**, 81.

Hakelius L. and Ponten B. (1973). Results of immediate and delayed surgical treatment of facial fractures with diplopia. *J. Maxillofac. Surg.*, **1**, 150.

Manson P.N., Clifford C.M., Iliff N.T., *et al*. (1986). Mechanisms of global support and post-traumatic enophthalmos. *Plast. Reconstr. Surg.*, **77**, 193.

Ord R.A. (1981). Postoperative retrobulbar haemorrhage and blindness complicating trauma surgery. *Br. J. Oral Surg.*, **19**, 202.

Perrott D.H. and Kaban L.B. (1993). Acute management of orbitozygomatic fractures. *Oral Maxillofac. Surg. Clin. North Am.*, **5**, 475.

Rowe N.L. and Williams J.Ll., eds (1985). *Maxillofacial Injuries* vol. 1. Edinburgh: Churchill Livingstone, chap. 12.

Chapter 9

Ophthalmic injuries

Ocular injuries associated with midfacial fractures

Al-Qurainy *et al*. (1991), in a prospective study in Glasgow involving 363 midfacial trauma patients over a 2 year period who were assessed by an ophthalmologist, found:

1. a. 90% of patients sustained ocular injuries
   b. 63% sustained minor injuries
   c. 16% moderate injuries
   d. 12% severe eye injuries
2. a. Severe ocular injuries most commonly seen in road traffic accidents (20%)
   b. Assaults had an 11% incidence of severe ocular injuries
3. Severe ocular trauma occurred in 33% of comminuted malar fractures and 17% of blowout fractures

Principal predictors which indicate the likelihood of underlying ocular trauma are: BAD ACT

1. **B**low-out fracture
2. **A**cuity
3. **D**iplopia
4. **A**mnesia
5. **C**omminuted **T**rauma

These predictors yield an efficient scoring system for detecting the risk of eye injury with a 90% specificity. This scoring system was developed in other papers by Al-Qurainy *et al*. (1991) based on 363 patients and was successfully tested on 100 patients in a further study.

Direct trauma to the globe

Blunt trauma to the eye

A sequence of injuries from front to back of eye:

1. Conjunctiva – oedema (chemosis)
   subconjunctival haemorrhage
2. Cornea – abrasion or laceration
3. Anterior chamber – bleeding from iris or ciliary body (hyphaema)
4. Iris – iridoplegia (fixed pupil)
   i. Traumatic miosis (constriction)
   ii. Traumatic mydriasis (dilatation)
   – iridodialysis (tear of iris)
5. Lens – dislocation
   traumatic cataract
6. Posterior chamber – vitreous haemorrhage caused by tear of the choroid
7. Retina – oedema – commotio retinae
   retinal haemorrhage
   detached retina – late complication
8. Optic nerve – optic atrophy leading to loss of vision
   nerve severed, e.g. orbital apex syndrome

Penetrating trauma to eye

1. Conjunctival laceration
2. Corneal laceration
3. Prolapse of iris through lacerated cornea
4. Perforation of lens
5. Perforation of choroid
6. Perforation of sclera
7. Foreign body

Treatment

Tetanus prophylaxis, eye pad, analgesics, refer to ophthalmologist for repair.

Injuries to specific structures

Eyelids

Laceration
Suture with 6/0 collagen, presume a lacerated globe until proven otherwise

Complications

1. Ectropion – eversion of eyelid with corneal exposure, this can be:
   a. Post-traumatic
   b. Post-surgical – blepharoplasty
   c. A result of facial nerve damage
2. Entropion – inversion of eyelid margin with abrasion of eyeball by inturned eyelashes

Conjunctiva

Damage to conjunctiva alone is rarely serious – subconjunctival haemorrhage, oedema and lacerations. Foreign bodies – evert upper or lower eyelid and remove foreign body with wet cotton bud. Use topical anaesthetic and fluorescein for easier identification.

Cornea

Abrasion, oedema, concussion necrosis, laceration – stain cornea with fluorescein for evidence of corneal abrasion. If present give antibiotic eyedrops.

Lacrimal apparatus

Injuries include:

1. Displacement of lower lacrimal punctum from surface of eye secondary to scar contracture or to avulsion of the medial canthal ligament – causes epiphora
2. Division of lacrimal canaliculus – related to tear of medial part of lower eyelid – causes epiphora
3. Damage related to nasomaxillary fractures, e.g. tear of lacrimal sac
4. Dacryocystitis – may result from tear in lacrimal sac causing inflammation and blockage of tears which may then become infected or enlarge to form a mucocoele – causes epiphora. Treated by dacryocystorhinostomy – fistulation of lacrimal sac into nose

Referral to ophthalmologist (Al-Qurainy *et al.*, 1991)

1. **Referral not necessary** – ocular injuries which recover spontaneously, e.g. orbital emphysema, conjunctival chemosis, sub-

conjunctival haemorrhage, corneal abrasion, periorbital bruising
2. **Routine referral** – ocular injuries for which non-urgent referral is indicated, e.g. enophthalmos, traumatic pupillary changes, conjunctival laceration, moderate reduction of visual acuity
3. **Early referral** – ocular injuries likely to lead to significant visual loss, e.g. retrobulbar haemorrhage, corneal damage, lens dislocation, severe reduction in visual acuity, optic nerve injury, retinal detachment

Management protocol

First priority is maintenance of vision and then restoration of appearance.

1. **Vision** – Assessment of visual acuity is important before and after facial surgery. Measured by reading fine print or using a Snellen chart at distance of 6 m. 6/6 is normal vision. Eyelids may have to be forced open to check vision. Assessment of pupillary light reflexes can give useful information regarding damage to optic nerve
2. **Loss of visual axis alignment** – Causes diplopia. Measured by Hess test

General rules

1. Do not remove or put anything in injured eye – just cover with light pad
2. Assume a laceration of eyelid means a damaged underlying globe until proven otherwise
3. Do not give topical anaesthetics for pain relief
4. Eye pain after facial surgery is usually of serious portent

Topical ophthalmic preparations

1. Antibiotics – 0.5% chloramphenicol eyedrops or 1% ointment
2. Local anaesthetic – amethocaine 1% eyedrops
3. Corneal stain – fluorescein – paper strips impregnated with 1 mg
4. Pupil dilator (mydriatic) – tropicamide 0.5% eyedrops
5. Pupil constrictor (miotic) – often used to reverse dilated pupil – pilocarpine 1%, 2% or 4% eyedrops

Diplopia

Stimulation of non-corresponding points of the two retinae by the same object.

Restriction of eye movement

1. Mechanical – e.g. trapping of extraocular muscle
2. Neurological – e.g. damage to nerve supply of extraocular muscles with a post-traumatic limitation of movement. Generally speaking the degree of diplopia caused by mechanical trapping of a muscle will be worst in the opposite direction of the field of action of affected muscle. It is the reverse for neurological damage

Incidence

Between 10% and 15% of middle third facial fractures. Al Qurainy *et al*. (1991) found a 20% incidence in 363 patients. Steidler *et al*. (1980) found a 32% incidence amongst middle-third fractures.

Principal risk factors

1. Blowout fractures (86% of cases had diplopia).
2. Road traffic accidents (31% had diplopia).
3. Comminuted malar fractures.

Types of diplopia

1. **Binocular diplopia** – far more common in traumatic injuries. In general terms in this situation the false *image* is projected in the same direction in which the trapped muscle normally moves the eye
2. **Monocular diplopia** – far less common.

Binocular diplopia (Rowe and Williams, 1985)

1. **Mechanical restriction of eye movement**
   a. Oedema, and/or extravasation of blood into and around extraocular muscles
   b. Muscle entrapment, e.g. inferior rectus in blowout fracture

   c. Fibrous adhesions – these usually develop some weeks after injury
   d. Trapping of periorbital fat in a bony defect
   e. Mechanical problems following displacement of one of the globes
2. **Neurological damage**
   a. Supranuclear lesions – contusion or compression of brain
   b. Nuclear lesions – contusion
   c. Damage to third, fourth and sixth cranial nerves
   d. Cavernous sinus thrombosis
   e. Superior orbital fissure syndrome

Monocular diplopia

This usually occurs with direct damage to globe:

- Detached retina
- Dislocation of the lens
- Damage to the macula

Assessment of diplopia

Difficult to assess in early stages because of oedema and periorbital bruising.

A. Diplopia test

Using linear light patient is questioned about separation of two images in cardinal positions of gaze. Greatest separation of images found in field of maximum limitation of movement.

B. Hess test

1. **Hess Screen** – divided into squares related to the cardinal positions of gaze there is an inner square of 9 dots and an outer square of 16 dots
2. **Test** – patient sits 50 cm from screen wearing glasses with one red and one green lens. Individual dots can be lit with a red light. Patient shines a green light from a torch on to the various positions where he sees the red light on the screen. The red and green glasses are reversed for testing the other eye

3. **Results** – a Hess Chart is plotted for each eye and the two fields are compared with each other and with the normal field printed on the chart
4. **Conclusions** – the plotted chart shows a restricted visual field and the tiny deviation in the primary position in the affected eye. It also shows a large field for the unaffected eye related to overaction of the muscle

Management of diplopia

Binocular diplopia

Most common cause is blowout fracture of orbit (see Chapter 8). When there is significant limitation of movement surgery is indicated in early stages. It should be noted that diplopia at extreme of upward gaze is not usually a problem unless patient is a pilot or billiard player.

Diplopia on downward gaze is a significant handicap with walking, reading, climbing ladders, etc.

Prognosis of diplopia

Prognosis of diplopia in blowout fractures of the orbit depends on:

1. Surgical technique
2. Time between injury and treatment
3. Degree of damage to muscles and their nerve supply
4. Orthoptic rehabilitation to achieve binocular single vision

Further reading

Al-Qurainy I.A., Stassen L.F.A., Dutton G.N. *et al*. (1991a). The characteristics of midfacial fractures and the association with ocular injury: a prospective study. *Br. J. Oral Maxillofac. Surg.*, **29**, 291.

Al-Qurainy I.A., Stassen L.F.A., Dutton G.N. *et al*. (1991b). Diplopia following midfacial fractures. *Br. J. Oral Maxillofac. Surg.*, **29**, 302.

Al-Qurainy I.A., Titterington D.M., Stassen L.F.A. *et al*. (1991c). Midfacial fractures and the eye: the development of a system for detecting patients at risk of eye injury. *Br. J. Oral Maxillofac. Surg.*, **29**, 363.

Al-Qurainy I.A., Dutton G.N., Ilankovan V., *et al*. (1991d). Midfacial fractures and the eye: the development of a system for detecting patients at risk of eye injury – a prospective evaluation. *Br. J. Oral Maxillofac. Surg.*, **29**, 368.

Culbertson W.W. (1983). Diagnosis and management of ocular injuries. *Otolaryngol. Clin. North Am.*, **16**, 563.
Duguid I.M. (1985). In *Maxillofacial Injuries* vol. II (Rowe N.L. and Williams J.Ll., eds). Edinburgh: Churchill Livingstone, chap. 16.
Holt G.R., Holt J.E. and Blodgett J.M. (1983). Ocular injuries during blunt facial trauma. *Ophthalmology*, **90**, 14.
Steidler N.E., Cook R.N. and Reade P.C. (1980). Residual complications in patients with major middle-third fractures. *Int. J. Oral Surg.*, **9**, 259.

Chapter 10

Nasal and nasoethmoidal injuries

Nasal injuries

Surgical anatomy

External nose

Upper part of nasal framework consists of two nasal bones together with the frontal processes of maxillae and nasal part of the frontal bone. Lower part of external nose consists of cartilaginous framework comprising septal cartilage, upper nasal cartilages and lower nasal cartilages.

Nasal septum

Perpendicular plate of ethmoid bone, vomer, septal cartilage.

Classification (Stranc and Robertson, 1979)

1. Frontal injuries:
   a. Plane 1 – lower end of nasal bone and anterior nasal spine
   b. Plane 2 – external nose
   c. Plane 3 – nasoethmoidal injury
2. Lateral injuries:
   a. Without septal fracture
   b. With septal fracture

External examination

- Nasal deformity
- Bruising and swelling
- Nasal bone crepitus

Intranasal examination (speculum and headlight)

- Clear debris and bloodclot
- Remove loose bone fragments
- Note any mucosal tears or damage to nasal septum

Timing of treatment

1. Preferably within first 24 hours post injury
2. Any time up to 7 days after injury

Treatment

Reduction
A. Closed manipulation
B. Submucous resection – deviation of septal cartilage
Immobilisation
C. Intranasal
- Ribbon gauze soaked in BIPP
- Silastic (silicone rubber wedges)
- Stainless steel intranasal splint (Sear, 1977)

D. External splint
- Plaster of Paris splint
- Collodion gauze and soft metal sheet
- Thermoplastic splint
- Lead compression plates

A. Closed manipulation

1. **Walsham's forceps** – left and right forceps to manipulate nasal bones at frontal process of maxillae
2. **Asche's septal forceps** – to iron out nasal septum and to elevate nasal bridge

Disadvantages

Studies have found that in nasal fractures treated by closed manipulation only 30% had normal appearance, and only 50% had normal function postoperatively. The problem with relapse appears to be related to immobilisation after reduction.

B. Submucous resection (SMR)

Harrison (1979) believes the SMR should be reserved for patients who exhibit airway obstruction due to distortion of septum. The buckled septal cartilage should be removed.

C. Intranasal immobilisation

1. **Ribbon gauze** – soaked in BIPP.
   Disadvantages:
   a. Obstructs airway and difficult to tolerate
   b. Potential infection – CSF rhinorrhea
   c. Overpacking causes telecanthus
2. **Silastic** – internally placed soft silicone wedges
3. **Stainless steel intranasal splint** – provides stable rigid internal nasal support

D. External fixation

1. **Plaster of Paris splint** – left in situ for 7–10 days, ideally should be replaced every 3–4 days as swelling subsides
2. **Gauze and soft metal sheet**:
   a. Several layers of cotton gauze soaked in collodion applied to nose and contoured
   b. Soft metal sheet (tin/lead alloy) cut to shape, applied and contoured
3. **Thermoplastic splint** – becomes malleable when heated and is adapted to nose
4. **Compression plates**
   a. Lead plates of 2 mm thickness with two holes drilled 1 cm apart
   b. Transnasal soft stainless steel wire 0.35 mm inserted as a horizontal mattress suture
   c. Lyofoam should be inserted between plates and surface of nose before tightening
   d. Transnasal wire should be removed after a few days – if left too long it will scar nasal skin
   e. Lead plates can be used in combination with anterior traction applied to an external skeletal frame

Nasoethmoidal injuries

Surgical anatomy

An area behind which lies the interorbital space which is situated between the medial walls of orbits. Fractures in this region are invariably comminuted.

Classification

Isolated nasoethmoidal injury

1. **Bilateral** – central midface injury resulting from direct blow over nasal bridge. Base of nose is driven backwards into interorbital space and nasal tip becomes upturned. Deep crease at base of nose and skin at base of nose frequently lacerated. CSF rhinorrhea should always be suspected
2. **Unilateral** – unilateral nasal deformity. Side of nose is depressed and there is underlying fracture of ethmoid bone

Combined nasoethmoid injury plus midface fractures

1. **Bilateral** – nasoethmoid complex fracture combined with Le Fort II and Le Fort III fractures. Causes traumatic telecanthus and elongation of midface
2. **Unilateral** – nasoethmoid complex injury plus severe comminution of orbit and zygomatic complex. Unilateral displacement of medial canthal ligament resulting in displacement of eye downwards and laterally

Clinical features

1. Frontal bone depression
2. Nasal deformity
3. Traumatic telecanthus
4. CSF fluid rhinorrhea
5. Diplopia
6. Haemorrhage from anterior or posterior branches of ethmoidal artery

Traumatic telecanthus

Increased intercanthal distance >35 mm (normal 25–35 mm) caused by:

1. Severance of canthi
2. Avulsion of canthi
3. Lateral displacement of medial canthal ligament whilst still attached to bone. May result in
   a. Narrow almond-shaped palpebral fissure
   b. More prominent epicanthal folds
   c. Diplopia

Treatment

A. Closed reduction

The use of transnasal wires and compression plates is often unsatisfactory.

B. Open reduction

Realignment of bony fragments under direct vision especially at early stages give better results.

Surgical approach

1. Existing laceration
2. H-shaped incision
3. Bilateral 'Z' incision
4. Midline vertical incision
5. W-shaped incision
6. Bicoronal flap
7. Degloving of nose plus bicoronal flap

Repair of bony skeleton

Nasal bridge re-attached to frontal bone. All bone fragments must be preserved, aligned and either directly wired or plated with microplates.

Medial canthal ligament

Surgical anatomy
Strong band of fibrous tissue which acts as tendon for origin of orbicularis muscle. Anterior part has a broad insertion to the anterior lacrimal crest. Posterior part passes behind lacrimal sac.

Repair
1. Once located the ligament must be repositioned and stabilised by direct transnasal wires
2. With severe comminution it may be necessary to place a bone graft in the area. Overcorrection of the telecanthus is desirable

Further reading

Banks P. (1987). *Killey's Fractures of the Middle Third of the Facial Skeleton*, 5th edn. Oxford: Butterworth Heinemann.

Bowerman J.E. (1985). In *Maxillofacial Injuries* vol. 1 (Rowe N.L. and Williams J.Ll., eds). Edinburgh: Churchill Livingstone, chap. 11.

Harrison D.H. (1979). Nasal Injuries – their pathogenesis and treatment. *Br. J. Plast. Surg.*, **32**, 57.

Sear A.J. (1977). A method of internal nasal splinting for unstable nasal fractures. *Br. J. Oral Surg.*, **14**, 203.

Stranc M.F. and Robertson G.A. (1979). A classification of injuries of the nasal skeleton. *Ann. Plast. Surg.*, **2**, 468.

Chapter 11

Gunshot injuries

Dynamics of gunshot injuries

Predominately young males:

- Military
- Civil violence
- Accidental
- Self inflicted

Physics of gunshot wounds

Wounding capacity depends on kinetic energy (KE) on impact

$KE = 1/2 \text{ mass} \times \text{velocity}^2$

Factors which affect the degree of injury include:

1. Velocity of bullet
2. Drag and retardation
3. Size of bullet
4. Composition and shape of bullet
5. Extent of cavitation which occurs
6. Extent of deformity or deviation (yaw) of bullet

Classification

Firearms

1. Low velocity	$<$ 1000 feet/second
2. High velocity	$>$ 1000 feet/second
4. Shotguns	$<$ 1000 feet/second

Gunshot wounds

1. **Penetrating wounds** – Low velocity projectile embedded in tissue with small point of entry

2. **Perforating wounds** – High velocity projectiles which pass right through tissues with exit wounds larger than entrance wounds
3. **Avulsive wounds** – Massive loss of tissue due to irregular fragments of shotgun pellets, bombs, grenades and mines travelling at medium velocity

Site of wound

1. **Tangential** – Cause peripheral damage to the face without involvement of cranial cavity
2. **Transverse**:
   a. High level – upper face involving eyes and cranial cavity, risk of meningitis
   b. Mid face – penetrating injuries to midface causing
      i. Oro-antral and oro-nasal communication
      ii. Severe epistaxis (anterior ethmoidal artery)
      iii. Ankylosis, related to comminution of coronoid process
   c. Lower face – loss of airway, feeding difficulties
   d. Neck – may lead to immediate exsanguination related to damage to major vessels in neck

Low velocity injuries

Injuries confined to bullet track, i.e. tissues are either lacerated or crushed. Small entry wounds with missile embedded in soft tissues. Injuries are not serious unless a vital organ or vessel is directly struck.

Shotgun injuries

Depends on distance of victim from shotgun:

1. **Close range (less than 10 feet)** – Central blast destroys areas of tissues which may clinically resemble a high velocity injury
2. **Long range** – Wounds consist of many small entry points of individual pellets. Invariably result in compound and comminuted bony fractures which are contaminated by foreign material and bacteria

High velocity injuries

Types of missiles

Soft nosed bullets
Civilian sporting rifles. Deform on impact to create large surface area resulting in wider track of destruction.

Hard nosed bullets
Military with complete copper jacket which usually pass through the body without changing shape.

Mechanisms of wounding

Shock waves
Injure surrounding tissues and are also conducted along blood vessels to distant sites.

Cavitation
Temporary expansion may be 40 times missile diameter before collapsing in pulsatile fashion resulting in massive tissue disruption. Thrombosis and stasis in vessels further increase extent of necrosis and oedema.

Secondary projectiles
When bullet strikes teeth or bone the energy is transferred to bony fragments which in turn become secondary projectiles accelerating in different directions.

Infection

Sources of contamination

1. Contaminated projectile
2. Material drawn into tissues from skin surface or clothes

Primary management of gunshot casualties

Immediate measures

- **A**irway
- **B**reathing
- **C**irculation
- Control of haemorrhage
- Analgesia

Transport to hospital

Documentation

- Date and time of injury
- Cause of injury

- Description of injury
- Immediate treatment given

Airway

Causes of obstruction

1. Haemorrhage
2. Foreign bodies
3. Prolapse of tongue
4. Oedema – in pharynx or larynx

First aid measures

1. Chin lift
2. Finger sweeps in mouth or suction
3. If airway and breathing established, turn into recovery position
4. If airway NOT established endotracheal intubation
5. Cricothyroidotomy in extreme emergency
6. Two large cannulae in peripheral veins – give Hartmann's solution
7. Control haemorrhage with pressure

Primary surgical management

Soft tissue wounds

Abundant blood supply of face usually allows primary closure without drainage after debridement. Gas gangrene of the face is extremely rare. Debridement and delayed primary closure with drainage is usual in other parts of the body when gross infection is present or wounds are more than 24 hours old.

Management of skin loss

1. **Primary closure** by undermining skin. Wound edges are excised and supported by subcutaneous sutures
2. **Dressing** to protect open wound and to allow epithelialisation from edges of wound
3. **Temporary suturing** of skin to mucosa to provide watertight seal and wound cover
4. **Split skin graft**

Low velocity injuries

Missile removed only if easily accessible since bullet becomes surrounded by fibrous tissue. Soft tissues heal spontaneously in this type of injury. For instance, if the entry and exit wounds are irrigated. Exploratory operation indicated where major vascular or organ injuries are suspected.

High velocity injuries

Extensive debridement may be necessary to deal with damaged tissues, well beyond the confines of the bullet track due to the widespread effects of shock waves and cavitation.

Injuries to facial skeleton

Basic surgical steps

1. **Debridement** – remove bullet fragments, fractured teeth, detached bone
2. **Closed reduction** – alignment of dental arches
3. **Suture of oral mucosa to skin**
4. **Drainage** – away from suture lines
5. **Postoperatively** – need special feeding

Features of bone fractures after gunshot wounds

1. Fractures are often comminuted and rarely produce a Le Fort injury
2. Minimal debridement and closed reduction to minimise interference with bone viability
3. Large oro-nasal or oro-antral fistulae may be created – pack with antiseptic gauze
4. Minimise likely residual defect during initial surgery to reduce functional loss and cosmetic deformity prior to secondary reconstruction

Secondary reconstructive surgery

Patient

A number of factors may influence the success of secondary surgery:

1. Age
2. Time since injury

3. General physical health
4. Psychological health

Secondary defects

Factors to be considered:

1. Alignment of bony structures
2. Alignment of soft tissues
3. Bone loss/soft tissue loss
4. Loss of specialised structures, e.g. eye, ear or nose
5. Scarring – site, extent
6. Special problems:
   a. Microstomia
   b. Temporomandibular joint ankylosis
   c. Oro-antral/oro-nasal fistulae
   d. Prosthetic rehabilitation

Planning reconstructive surgery

1. Removal of foreign bodies
2. Release of scar contractures
3. Re-establishment of bony framework – including bone grafting
4. Reconstruction of damaged nerves
5. Closure of fistulae
6. Soft tissue coverage:
   a. Skin grafts
   b. Local and distant flaps
   c. Revision of scars – Z- or W-plasty where scars lie across lines of skin tension
7. Special considerations of the face:
   a. Lacrimal apparatus
   b. Facial nerve
   c. Parotid ducts
   d. Commissures of mouth
   e. Canthi of eyes

Further reading

Awty M.D. and Banks P. (1971). Treatment of maxillofacial casualties in the Nigerian Civil War. *Oral Surg. Oral Med. Oral Pathol.*, **31**, 4.

Banks P. (1985). In *Maxillofacial Injuries*, vol. II, (Rowe N.L. and Williams J.Ll., eds), Edinburgh, Churchill Livingstone, chap. 14.

Irby W.B. (1969). Facial Injuries in military combat: intermediate care. *J. Oral. Surg.*, **27**, 548.

Chapter 12

Head injuries

Scalp injuries

Anatomy

Five layers (Figure 12.1)

1. Skin
2. Subcutaneous tissues
3. Galea aponeurotica
4. Loose areolar tissue
5. Periosteum (pericranium)

Injuries and treatment

Simple lacerations

- Debridement and suture
  Galea 3/0 catgut
  Skin 3/0 nylon, or staples

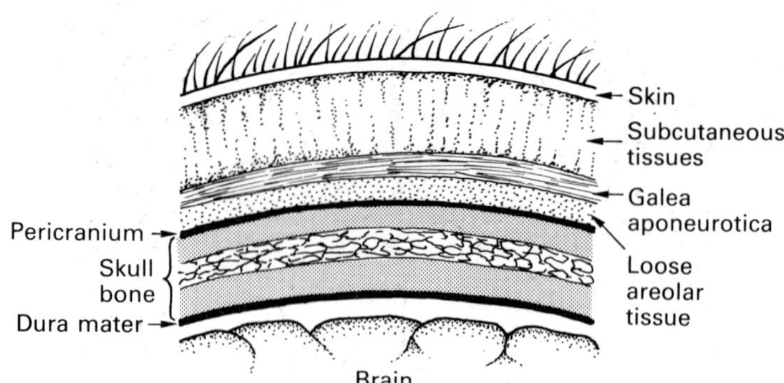

Figure 12.1 Layers of scalp and skull.

Scalp loss

- Intact periosteum and skull
  - Split thickness grafts
- Destroyed periosteum and skull fracture
  - Local flaps
  - Distant flaps
- Microvascular reattachment

Types of head injury

1. Skull fractures (Figure 12.2)

Significance of skull fracture is that it identifies patient with a high probability of developing an intracranial haematoma.

A. Linear non-depressed fractures
Usually no treatment required. Fractures across artery, e.g. middle meningeal should raise suspicion of extradural haemorrhage.

B. Depressed skull fractures
May be neurosurgical emergency. To reduce future risks, e.g. epilepsy, any fragment depressed more than thickness of skull requires elevation of bony fragment.

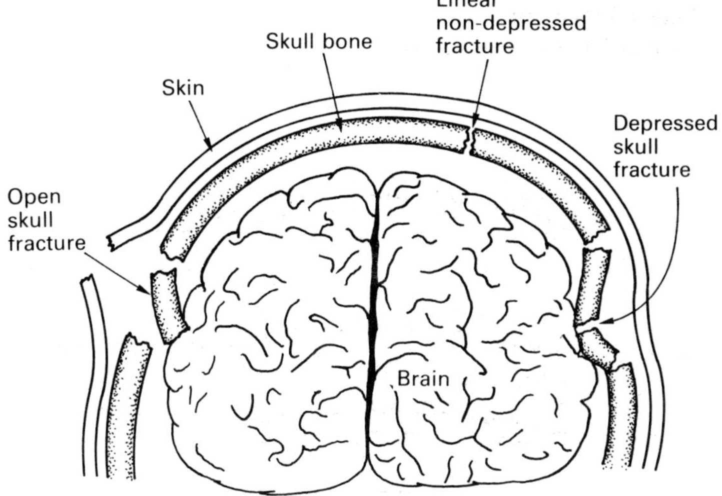

Figure 12.2 Types of skull fractures.

C. Open skull fractures
Communication between scalp laceration and the brain. Diagnosed if brain visible or CSF is leaking from wound. May require early operative intervention with closure of dura.

D. Base of skull fractures
Usually not seen on skull X-rays. Diagnosis based on clinical examination, e.g. CSF leaking from ear (otorrhea) or nose (rhinorrhea). Bruising in mastoid region (Battle's sign) indicates base of skull fracture as does blood behind tympanic membrane (haemotympanum). Cribriform plate fractures often associated with periorbital bruising (Panda facies).

Primary treatment

Skull fractures
- Removal or elevation of bone
- Fixation of bone with plates or wires

Tears of dura mater
Repaired by:
1. Direct closure
2. Pericranial graft
3. Autogenous fascia lata
4. Zenoderm (freeze-dried porcine skin)

Secondary repair

Indications
1. Vulnerable to trauma
2. Poor aesthetics
3. Patient concerned – pulsatile headache
4. Soft head

Methods
1. Bone grafts:
   a. Split rib grafts
   b. Iliac crest
2. Metallic plates:
   Titanium
3. Acrylic implants

2. Diffuse brain injuries

Occur when rapid head motions (acceleration or deceleration) cause widespread damage to brain.

A. Concussion

Head injury causing brief loss of neurological functions. Causes temporary confusion or amnesia. Patient may complain of nausea, dizziness, headache. If patient has been knocked unconscious, should be admitted for 24 hours of neurological observations.

B. Diffuse axonal injury (DAI)

Microscopic structural damage throughout brain. Causes prolonged coma lasting days or weeks. Mortality about 33%. Diagnosis made by CT scan when no mass lesion is present. These patients require long-term coma care.

3. Focal injuries

Local area of macroscopic damage. These can be contusions, haemorrhages or haematomas. Because of their mass effects they may require emergency treatment. This group of injuries frequently requires emergency surgery.

A. Contusion

Cerebral contusion. Serious concussions with prolonged coma and confusion. Contusions can occur at point of impact (coup contusions) or can occur on opposite side of head (contrecoup contusions). A CT scan will determine the presence, site and size of a contusion.

B. Intracranial haemorrhages

Meningeal haemorrhages

1. **Extradural haemorrhage** (Figure 12.3) – Caused by tear in dural artery, e.g. middle meningeal artery. Fairly rare injury – 0.9% of unconscious head injuries. Often a linear skull fracture over artery is present. Signs and symptoms include:
   a. Loss of consciousness

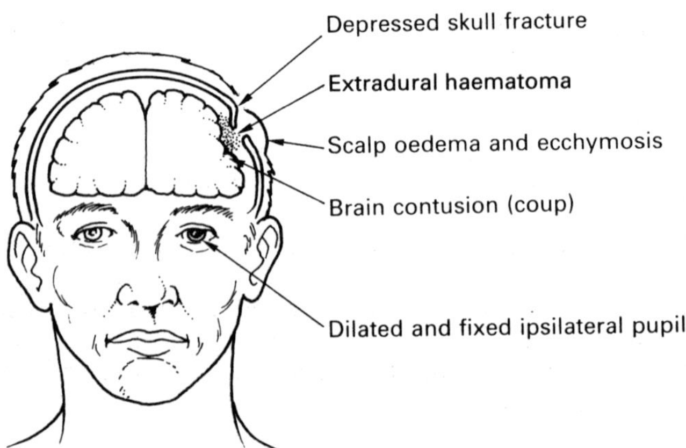

Figure 12.3 Extradural haemorrhage.

b. Intervening lucid period
c. Secondary depressed consciousness
d. Development of hemiparesis on opposite side. A fixed dilated pupil occurs on same side as injury This requires emergency surgery. Prognosis is usually excellent.

2. **Subdural haemorrhage** (Figure 12.4) – Occurs in 30% of head injuries. Usually caused by tearing of bridging veins between brain and dura mater. Prognosis poor and mortality 60%. Requires emergency surgery.
3. **Subarachnoid haemorrhage** – Causes blood-stained CSF.

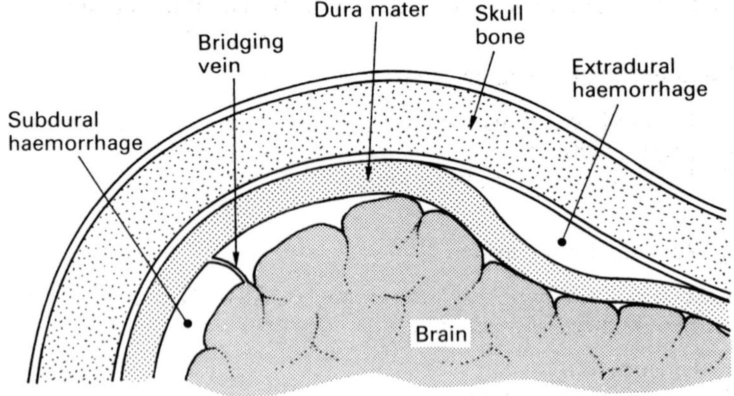

Figure 12.4 Diagram showing extradural and subdural haemorrhages.

Meningeal irritation causing headache and photophobia. Emergency surgery not needed. CT scan clinches diagnosis

Brain haemorrhages and lacerations

1. **Intracerebral haematoma** – Diagnosed by CT scan. Hemiplegia may occur. Bleeding into ventricles and cerebellum, has a high mortality rate
2. **Impalement injuries** – Foreign bodies protruding from or traversing skull should be left in place. X-rays of skull are required and objects should be removed by neurosurgeons
3. **Bullet wounds** – The lower the bullet in the brain the worse the prognosis. Extent of damage related to size and velocity of bullet (see Chapter 11)

Assessment of head injuries

History

Type of injury

A head injury caused by a fall is four times as likely to have an intracranial haematoma than a road traffic accident. Assessment by ambulance staff can give important information as to whether patient is deteriorating.

Vital signs

Airway, breathing and control of circulation *must* take priority. Failure to take these basic steps will increase brain damage.

Minineurological examination

A. Level of consciousness
B. Pupil reactions
C. Lateralised extremity weakness

A. Level of consciousness

Assessed by Glasgow Coma Scale (GCS). This is the sum of scores for three assessments:

1. Eye opening
2. Best motor response
3. Verbal Response

1. **Eye opening (E score)** – valid if patient's eyes can be opened
   a. Spontaneous – eyes open with normal blinking
      E = 4 points
   b. Speech – responds to request for eye opening
      E = 3 points
   c. Pain – eye opens with painful stimulus
      E = 2 points
   d. No eye opening
      E = 1 point
2. **Best motor response (M score)**
   a. Obeys – moves limbs when requested
      M = 6 points
   b. Localises – purposeful movement towards painful stimulus
      M = 5 points
   c. Withdraws – pulls away from painful stimulus
      M = 4 points
   d. Abnormal flexion – decorticate posture
      M = 3 points
   e. Extension response – decerebrate posture
      M = 2 points
   f. No movement
      M = 1 point
3. **Verbal response (V score)** – not possible if patient intubated
   a. Orientated in time and place
      V = 5 points
   b. Confused conversations – answers questions
      V = 4 points
   c. Inappropriate words – clear words but inappropriate use
      V = 3 points
   d. Sounds only – grunts and groans
      V = 2 points
   e. No verbal response
      V = 1 point

The Glasgow Coma Scale is used to categorise patients:

Coma No eye opening E = 1
No ability to follow commands M = 1–5
No verbal response V = 1 or 2

Patients with a Glasgow Coma Score of 8 or less are in coma

Severity of head injury

i. Severe head injury – if GCS is equal to or less than 8

ii. Moderate head injury – GCS 9–12
iii. Minor head injury – GCS 13–15

B. Pupil reactions

A difference in pupil diameters or more than 1 mm is abnormal. Sluggish light reflex may indicate an intracranial injury. A fixed dilated pupil indicates considerably raised intracranial pressure.

C. Lateralised extremity weakness

Spontaneous movements are observed. If no spontaneous movement try painful stimulus. Delayed or reduced movement compared with other side indicates lateralised extremity weakness.

Investigations

A. Computerised tomography

A CT scan is the single most important investigation.

B. Skull X-rays

Of limited value in patient with obvious head injury.

Management of head injuries

Once a provisional diagnosis has been made, treatment should be aimed at protecting the brain from secondary injury.

A. Maintenance of cerebral metabolism
B. Prevention or treatment of intracranial hypertension

A. Maintenance of cerebral metabolism

Main metabolic requirements of brain are oxygen and glucose. Glucose is usually not a problem. Oxygen concentration can be assessed by blood gases and oxygen can be given. Blood transfusion may be necessary. A good cerebral blood flow is dependent on systemic arterial pressure and the arterial $P\text{CO}_2$. Control of blood pressure and maintenance of $P\text{CO}_2$ at 26–28 mmHg maintains adequate cerebral blood flow.

B. Preventing or treating intracranial hypertension

Intracranial hypertension may be due to a mass lesion, acute brain swelling or oedema of the brain. Treatment includes:

1. **Induced hypocapnia** – lowering of $P\text{CO}_2$ in cerebral vessels causes vasoconstriction and reduces intracranial pressure. Hyperventilation is induced to reduce the arterial $P\text{CO}_2$ to a range of 26–28 mmHg. Intubation of trachea required with paralysis. Blood gases must be monitored
2. **Fluid control** – judicious administration of fluids to prevent overhydration
3. **Diuretics** – mannitol can shrink the brain by producing an intravascular hyperosmolarity. Loop diuretics such as frusemide may help
4. **Steroids** – the efficacy of steroids is questionable

Surgical management of head injuries

Essential diagnostic studies should be completed within 2 hours of injury. Surgical treatment should be carried out by a neurosurgeon. Surgery in particular is aimed at dealing with mass lesions or skull fractures. Any haematoma is evacuated. The dura mater is repaired and bone fragments are replaced and fixed.

Care of the unconscious patient

1. **Airway**
   a. Oral/nasal tube
   b. Endotracheal tube
   c. Tracheostomy
2. **Fluids, electrolytes, nutrition**
   a. Intravenous
   b. Nasograstric
3. **Bladder, bowels, bedsores**
4. **Temperature regulation**
   a. Damaged hypothalamus
   b. Increased body temperature – increased cerebral oedema and oxygen requirements
5. **Treatment**
   a. Aspirin
   b. Promethazine 25–50 mg i.m.
   c. Tepid sponging
   d. Fans/icepacks

Complications of head injuries

Post-concussional syndrome

Memory loss, confusion and disorientation. Residual problems depend on degree of initial injury. Patient may have persistent headaches, loss of balance and co-ordination. Takes 1–3 years to return to normal.

Post-traumatic amnesia

When it exceeds 1 week personality and intellectual disturbances are common.

Post-traumatic epilepsy

Risk of developing epilepsy:

- Mild injury = 2%
- Post-traumatic amnesia > 24 hours = 10%
- Intracranial haematoma = 30%
- Cortical laceration = 50%

Risk becomes negligible (assuming no fits) after 5 years.
Prophylactic anti-convulsent therapy required for:

- Depressed fracture of skull
- Acute intracranial haematoma

Brain death

When to consider the possibility of brain death

- Coma
- Requirement for artificial ventilation
- Serious diagnosis, e.g. intracerebral haemorrhage

Test to confirm brain death

- Fixed pupils
- Oculo-vestibular reflex absent
- Corneal reflex absent
- No motor cranial response
- No gag reflex
- No spontaneous respirations after discontinuing intermittent positive pressure ventilation (IPPV)

When to withdraw treatment

Two independent senior neurologists should examine patient 30 minutes apart, at least 6 hours after injury.

Cerebrospinal fluid leaks

Pathology

An abnormal communication between the meninges and the extracranial spaces such as the paranasal sinuses resulting from a tear in the dura mater.

1. **Occurrence** – Suspect the possibility of CSF leak with all high level facial fractures and base of skull fractures.
2. **Sites**
   a. Nose – rhinorrhoea
   b. Ears – otorrhoea

Clinical presentation

1. High level facial fractures, e.g. nasoethomoidal, Le Fort II and III
2. Base of skull fractures, e.g. petrous temporal bone

Management

1. Prophylactic antibiotics. Most CSF leaks cease spontaneously after a few days, especially after maxillary fractures have been reduced and fixed
2. Surgical repair of dural breach:
   a. Possible indications for surgical intervention
      i. CSF leak > 10 days
      ii. Recurrent CSF leak
      iii. Meningitis
   b. Possible timing of repair
      i. Early – at time of reduction of facial bones
      ii. Late – after reduction of facial bones

Complications of CSF leaks

1. Fistula formation with significant CSF loss
2. Ascending infection – meningitis
3. Aerocoele
4. Death

Further reading

Cantore G.P. *et al*. (1979). Cranio-orbital-facial injuries. *J. Trauma*, **19**, 370.

Chandler J.R. (1983). Traumatic cerebrospinal leakage. *Otolaryngol. Clin. North Am.*, **16**, 623.

Committee on Trauma, American College of Surgeons (1988). *Advanced Trauma Life Support Student Manual* American College of Surgeons: *Head Trauma*, chap. 6.

Jennett B. and Teasdale G. (1981). *Management of Head Injuries*. Philadelphia: F.A. Davis.

Leopard P.J. (1971). Dural tears in maxillofacial injuries. *Br. J. Oral. Surg.*, **8**, 222.

McKusick K.A. (1977). The diagnosis of traumatic cerebrospinal rhinorrhea. *J. Nucl. Med.*, **18**, 1234.

Teasdale G. and Jennett B. (1974). Assessment of coma and impaired consciousness: a practical scale. *Lancet*, **ii**, 81.

Index

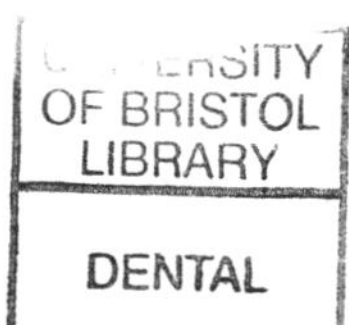